MW00914530

"Life is too important to be lived haphazardly. *Life's Third Act* explains through vivid examples what growing older is really like. The author's illustrations show how change and loss can lead to new opportunities, even joy, for those prepared to manage their own lives during key periods of transition."

—Gerald G. Garbacz, chairman and CEO, Baker & Taylor

"Our society faces new public issues because of the increasing proportion of our population who are over the age of 50. Unfortunately, many are unprepared for the types of changes we typically experience as we age. In *Life's Third Act,* Pat Burnham emphasizes the importance of planning each time new circumstances occur in our lives. This readable book illustrates that most of us should and can be responsible for ourselves, rather than expecting others to take care of these matters."

—Kay Orr, former governor of Nebraska

"Reading *Life's Third Act* made me talk with my wife about the decisions and changes we will have to make next in our lives. Pat Burnham deals honestly with aging and, better yet, presents the opportunities which can come with the freedom of our mature years. We will buy copies for each of our four children so they will better understand what we will be experiencing in the years ahead."

—John Downs, lawyer and writer, Downs, Rachlin & Martin

"What a good idea this book has! So many of my patients slide toward aging and death with little sense of how to plan and how to choose. These stories bring to life ways of choosing. And, unlike our culture, where death is shunned and unacknowledged, this book looks squarely at decline and death and gives us strong leadership in meeting the related difficulties. I hope my patients read it."

—Dr. Tim Thompson, family physician

"Pat Burnham handles transitions with skill and sensitivity. In *Life's Third Act,* she also demonstrates her effectiveness in communicating with a diverse audience about a subject many of us like to avoid—our own aging. Her compelling stories about growing older will motivate men and women over 50 to manage their own lives with greater satisfaction. This book should be in every library."

—Beth Mason, reference librarian, Wilton, Connecticut

"The author of *Life's Third Act* has considerable experience with adult development and transition management. Dr. Burnham effectively translates research findings into believable stories and clear concepts from which readers can learn about controlling the transitions in their own lives. I highly recommend this book for your personal library."

—Dent Rhodes, professor of education, Illinois State University

"As I work with executives in major corporations and institutions, I am keenly aware of the personal issues that develop as a result of job-related changes. Pat Burnham brings her management experience in both the corporate and nonprofit worlds to this sound and easily read book, which offers excellent material for either family discussions, or retirement planning seminars intended to assist people in making decisions about how to live once they leave full-time employment."

—Douglass Lind, Ph.D., corporate advisor and therapist

LIFE'S THIRD ACT

TAKING CONTROL
OF YOUR MATURE YEARS

Patricia W. Burnham, Ph.D.

Patricia W. Burnham, 1995

With love and appreciation
for your special experiences
with transitions —

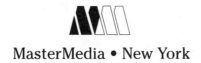

MasterMedia • New York

Published 1994 by MasterMedia Limited

MASTERMEDIA and colophon are registered trademarks
of MasterMedia Limited

Library of Congress Cataloging-in-Publication Data

Burnham, Patricia W.
    Life's third act : taking control of your mature years / Patricia W. Burnham
        p.   cm.
    Includes biological references.
    ISBN 1-57101-003-3 (hardbound) : $18.95
    1. Middle-aged persons—United States—Life skill guides.
2. Aged—United States—Life skill guides.   I. Title.
HQ1059.5.U5B87 1994
305.24'4—dc20   94-3066

Manufactured in the United States of America
Book design by Alan L. Marks
Production services by Lynn & Turek Associates, New York

10 9 8 7 6 5 4 3 2 1

To

Bob,
my beloved and ever challenging partner
in life's third act

~

Cinda, Chris, and Duncan,
that they may better understand
their own changing roles
in the drama of their mother's life

~

the memory of my parents' patience
when I failed to recognize that their aging years
held both joyous and painful scenes.

Contents

Contents

Foreword

As long as I can remember, I have recognized choice as the measure of human privilege. Those with choices of food and drink, of clothing and shelter, of work and entertainment, are the fortunate, the privileged ones. I believe that privilege can be measured by the quantity and quality of the choices available to us. We can acquire choices collectively through membership in a powerful tribe or social class, or individually through our professional, political, or economic position. The privilege of choice can be bestowed or it can be earned—and it can be taken away.

The vital message of this book is that retirement or, as a friend of mine describes it, "getting nearer the end of the pipeline," need not—indeed, should not—take this privilege away. What more hopeful message can there be for all us? I say "all" because all of us are moving in one direction along that pipeline and caring about someone else farther along than ourselves.

"Taking control" means, to me, exerting the privilege of choice. I believe that those who speak of taking control of our lives recognize that there is no such option as absolute control: accidents and health crises, acts of God and war can intervene. But the urge to take control of at least something, no matter how great the constraints imposed by nature or society, must be central to what is human—throughout the pipeline.

My infant granddaughter, her brain developing, struggles to control her muscles and limbs to touch things and stand up. My husband, his brain deteriorating, also struggles to control his limbs to touch things and stand up. Theirs is a physical struggle for control, but I know that my husband has the conscious choice of whether or not to try: he chooses to try, and feels better about himself by doing so. And we all know the proud smile of the infant when she does manage to touch something she wants. Both young and old, vigorous and ill, struggle to assert the right to make choices, and then relish in making them.

Why is choice so vital? I think we all know why. It makes us feel that we have some power, some identity, some meaning in the cosmos. Isn't one of the pleasures of going out for dinner to choose from a menu? When we choose a car, a home, a Christmas present, aren't we saying "Look at me, I know what I'm doing, I am in control!" (Is this one reason why women, in less powerful positions than men, love to shop?) These choices are more than those of the infant or infirm for physical control. They are cognitive choices between alternatives that reflect the values, the culture, and the experiences that define us as individuals. Choice of the red sports car over the black sedan tells us as much about the needs and values of the chooser as does the choice of the low cholesterol meal over the steak. Through the choices made by the individuals whose stories are told in this book, Patricia Burnham illuminates their beliefs, their culture—their very personhood.

Our personal and cultural values are central to how we use the privilege of our choices. These, in turn, are a product of our heritage, prejudices, ideals, habits, experiences, religion, and politics. I have felt the least choice during the sixty-six years of my life when I assumed that the birth accident of being female predetermined big choices for me. Time and again I have resented responsibilities I felt I was "stuck" with because I was female and "had to" assume the woman's role. Why did I have to do it at all? Why was I the only one to take care of my mother, my husband, and the one to provide ninety percent of the care of my sons? Males with the professional skills and responsibilities that I had, did not have to "do it all." Now, I recognize that I did have a choice: determined by my needs and values and influenced by assumptions about my cultural role as female.

I placed a high value on and needed the caregiving and companionship I saw in other homes, because I had missed them in mine. I wanted to be the best mother and wife possible. At the same time I loved the intellectual adventures and collegiality of science, but perhaps had less need than others to make it my top priority because I had already belonged to the scientific community through my father, and had grown up surrounded by happy, successful scientists. As evidence of the values that conditioned my choices then, I remember saying that I never wanted to tell my sons, "Don't bother Mother, she's thinking." Doing beautiful science would have required such concentration—an entirely valid choice for some, but apparently not for me. Other women, with different priorities, chose a different balance between home and work.

I chose an adaptable daytime educational job that left long evenings and holidays free for family life. Although I partly resented my male colleagues for not having to face such a decision, I now recognize that having such a choice was a privilege that many men would envy! In the stories that follow, male, female, and family roles often were taken for granted, and yet those who did take control often did so by reversing roles. As men are now allowed to shed some of the formerly required "macho" mantle, we are finding that many men relish, and are good at, full-time caregiving. Others resent it. Watching our friends in their "golden years," I notice one thing critical to their success is whether the husband welcomes or resents his release from breadwinning roles.

Cultural values do change. Our disastrous AIDS epidemic is bringing "out of the closet" the caring and commitment of men as caregivers. Even when this epidemic fades from the news, my guess is that the role of caregiver, male or female, will remain freshly valued. Vividly do I remember the words of a professional colleague on dealing with the changing youth culture of the '60s. Her husband had been a beautiful father, husband, and musician who died too young through his inability to deal also with society's expectation that he must be the chief breadwinner in the family. My friend expressed the most profound regret that her husband had not lived long enough to take advantage of the changing mores of male and female roles.

Taking control by making choices opens doors to unpredictable and unplanned-for possibilities that may even make you feel less in control! First juggling children and job, and then job and community and cause-related activities, I discovered that I had chosen to keep many balls in the air rather than concentrate on virtuosity with one. The balls kept bouncing into uncharted territories, places I now am grateful I was able to explore. Through invitations to serve on the boards of directors of four companies, I became one of a handful of academics who have been able to learn about and contribute to corporate enterprise. Knowing about the world of business from the inside certainly makes me a more useful educator—and grandmother! And my knowledge of science and technology has contributed, in unexpected ways, to my directorships. Elected as the first woman to join Avon Products' Board of Directors (there are now five of us!), my experience as a woman manager was what attracted the board to me. What they got, in addition, was a former scientist whose research on skin was already in textbooks and the *Journal of Cosmetic Chemists!* A bonus for us both, as it turned out.

The one choice we do not have is to be immortal!

Mortality robs us of choice: sometimes all at once, and sometimes bit by bit. A good friend turned to me recently to say how sad she was that my husband was in a nursing home. I tried to tell her that the tragedy was not the nursing home, but his mortality, his progressive debilitation. His skilled nursing facility is a blessing. It offers us choice. Living there allows him to have more control of his life than would be possible if he was being nursed in a small city apartment or isolated country home.

Illness, pain, and loss of physical control is the tragedy, not the institutions and caregivers who choose to help us. As I am once again a caregiver, spending much time with bright, skilled, and caring nurses and other caregivers, I have found humanity to be our final choice. To be humane and caring is a choice. As a society, as relatives, as nurses we can still choose whether or not to be compassionate and express sisterly love. The love and compassion of humanity can take over control when choice recedes.

—*Cecily Cannan Selby, Ph.D.*

Preface

*"For age is opportunity no less
than youth itself."*

—HENRY WADSWORTH LONGFELLOW

Life's Third Act: Taking Control of Your Mature Years is a product of my own search for meaning as I approached age 60. Consequently, this book is based on personal experience—as wife, mother, educator, corporate manager, and international business consultant. The composite characters presented here are based on the stories of people I have interviewed, although none is intended to portray any specific person I know. What you read here is also grounded in considerable research of the current literature on aging that has developed within several different professional fields—gerontology, social work, nursing, counseling, adult development, philosophy, religion, and financial planning.

While these categories seem to be somewhat nonparallel, they reflect the diverse descriptors under which I have located the literature on growing older in both academic and community libraries, as well as in bookstores. In one major Manhattan bookstore, you have to work your way through several crowded rooms to a distant corner near the fire exit in order to find the shelf titled "Aging." Apparently, some people are uncomfortable with this topic, and almost no one is quite sure what this broad subject of growing older includes or where it fits!

As I passed my mid-fifties, I realized that I was becoming impatient with my various title-defined corporate and community roles. At this point, our children were away from home and, theoretically, financially independent. My husband was making the transition from being a university administrator to being a professor. My father and step-mother lived many miles away, and their needs and desires were both increasing and unpredictable. Profes-sionally, I was consulting extensively with two Japanese companies who seemed to value my accessibility and quick responsiveness as much as they did my ideas. This combination of circumstances resulted in my feeling busy and pressured, but not very fulfilled.

Since I had not quite decided that I had a problem, I certainly could not define it clearly. And, because I could not clearly define my concerns, I was not in a position to receive much help or support from others. My attempts to talk with friends or advisors about some of these matters resulted in their concluding that I was either "burned out" with a specific activity or organization or that I just wanted to "take life easier" at this age. Neither was correct, and I recognized it, although I could not explain what I did mean. Fortunately, my husband and I openly shared our feelings about the present and our concerns for the future during this period.

Gradually, I began to seek out people older than I whose lives seemed vital and interesting, even though I already knew that most had experienced losses as well. I also talked with men and women in my age range whom I knew to have concerns for their parents, adult children, careers, and community roles. These discussions were, at first, informal. Later, I conducted a series of structured interviews with both individuals and couples in order to focus on their attitudes toward and experiences with aging.

While my own career roles have been varied, the most

significant theme of my work has been the development of people through the transitions of their lives. Now, I sought to bring up-to-date my reading of both fiction and nonfiction books and articles about adult transitions and the search for meaning. This broad approach led me to materials as diverse as those on the representative list, titled "Resources," included with this book. While my research was largely complete by the time the books by Jack and Phoebe Ballard, Deepak Chopra, Betty Friedan, and Tracy Kidder became available in the latter months of 1993, I find them complementary to my own work and, therefore, include them here for your reference.

As my personal exploration, the series of interviews, and my library research proceeded, I also became more deeply acquainted with aging issues through the changes being experienced by my father and stepmother. My mother had died a number of years ago, and I realize now that I did not take the time I needed to grieve that loss. Recently, I have struggled not only to find ways to assist my father while preserving his sense of independence and self-worth, but also to accept the fact that I never fully valued the man he once was. I have also had to recognize my lost opportunities—and those of my children and grandchildren—to plan a future that includes him. In spite of these disappointments and frustrations, my father and I established a closer, more loving relationship during his final months than we had previously had. His death on January 22, 1994, before he could actually touch the reality of this book of which he was so much a part, came more quickly than we had expected. I suppose that death usually does come too quickly, even as we are relieved that pain and loss have ended for a loved one.

During my personal explorations and research, I decided to share with others some of these insights about growing older and my ideas for handling the many transitions we face through this book. I selected the title, *Life's Third Act*, because in dramatic literature this act usually represents the most important and exciting part of the production. In Act III the principal characters reach full development and act out the most significant scenes of the entire plot.

I honestly believe that the period after my mid-fifties is the most exciting and interesting period of my life. There is every reason to believe that there will be many scenes ahead, each offering new settings, roles, and plot twists. Like Thomas A. Edison. "I am long on ideas, but short on time. I expect to live to be only a hundred." The fact that I will die at the end of the Third Act does not change my belief or diminish the excitement. After all, even the best dramatic performances must have a final curtain! I certainly do not want to be on stage forever, although I intend to make every scene in my life as joyful and productive as I possibly can.

The purpose of this book is to present through personal stories the typical changes faced by people after age 50 and to provide guidelines for making personal transitions gracefully, with control and dignity. Chapter 1, *Purposeful Aging*, introduces the topic of aging and the context in which we grow older in the last decade of the twentieth century.

Chapter 2, *Productive Scenes or Unresolved Crises*, introduces some typical joys and losses of the early decades of aging as experienced in the lives of three different couples. We become acquainted with the problems and decisions, as well as the new possibilities, that begin to confront persons as early as age 50 and typically develop by age 75.

Chapter 3, *Role Changes Under Pressure*, tells the stories of two sets of people in their late seventies. It portrays some of the pleasures and losses that prompt additional decisions to manage the transitions required of many in the latter years of life.

Chapter 4, *Culminating Scenes*, describes some of the difficult loss issues that octogenarians often face and their possible responses to these circumstances as seen through the lives of a widowed man and a couple who married each other after their previous spouses died.

Chapter 5, *Planning the Next Scenes*, introduces the concept of mature planning and decision-making as a series of steps that we each need to take repeatedly in sequential periods of life. Using the case studies and composite characters first presented in chapters 2 through 4, we observe how women and men make transitions and examine our common needs for challenge, commitment, and control.

Chapter 6, *Taking Control Strategies for Transitions*, explains through narrative and graphic models the common strategies that can be effective in dealing with new challenges during your aging years. This chapter also offers examples of how the strategies might be applied to addressing typical planning tasks.

Chapter 7, *Outstanding Performances*, presents brief examples of persons whose lives have exhibited strength or regeneration in their mature years and summarizes the key themes in this book. Finally, this chapter challenges each of us to use tested planning strategies to assure that our own aging years will be filled with joy and productivity according to our own measure.

Pablo Casals, the famed cellist, at age 96, said to a concert audience, "I am an old man, but in many senses a very young man. And this is what I want you to be, young, young all your life, and to say things to the world that are true." Like Casals, I want to have worthwhile challenges and purposeful commitments and be in control of my life—qualities we associate with the young—and I want to tell you about what I believe to be true about maintaining those qualities as we age.

Patricia W. Burnham
East Burke, Vermont

Purposeful Aging

CHAPTER ONE

*"Every age has its pleasures, its style
of wit, and its own ways."*

—Nicolas Bouleau Despreaux

IMPROVISING OUR AGING

Those of us growing older in our society are gaining in numbers and public attention. While aging may not be fashionable in all circles, more of us live longer than our parents and grandparents did, more of us stay physically active, and many have the mental health and economic resources necessary to take on challenging new tasks and move in new directions. Aging minorities have the same financial, health, and family issues as others, but may also face additional challenges, such as language, cultural confusion about roles, militancy of their young, or general prejudice. Research indicates that people of all racial and ethnic groups can grow in knowledge and understanding, learn new physical skills, and be sexually active well into their 70s and 80s, even if some prefer less strenuous activities part of the time.

We live in a society which has not prepared for us and which seems to lack adequate role models or examples for dynamic living in the years after age 50. We need to use our experience and energy in ways which seem productive and satisfying. It's as if we have to improvise our roles and scripts for playing out this act of our lives.

While some would have us move quietly and predictably toward patterns of behavior which customarily are regarded as "appropriate" for the elderly, that scenario does not suit most of us. In the past, Western society has expected those of us over 50 to engage in activities deemed suitable to the aging, to be content with our status, to be uncomplaining and undemanding—even submissive—and to have enough happiness and peacefulness to share with a harried younger populace.

Few literary, film, or television presentations include well developed characterizations of aging people leading active and interesting lives. Quotations about the old or aging tend to be negative, although there are some inspiring or entertaining exceptions. I like George Burns' question, "How can I die? I'm booked." Or Gypsy Rose Lee's famous comment, "I have everything now I had 20 years ago—except now it's all lower." On the inspiring side, we can appreciate John Donne's lines, "No spring, nor summer beauty hath such grace, As I have seen in one autumnal face." And, we are moved by Will Durant's tribute, "The love we have in our youth is superficial compared to the love that an old man has for his old wife."

We over age 50 are clearly becoming a powerful group politically, as our concerns for healthcare and insistence on opportunities for real choices in lifestyle demonstrate. Regrettably, not all of the changing conditions in society have positive implications for the aging. While more people live longer than ever before, some live for years after their income, or health, fails. The major family "breadwinner" is apt to retire earlier than before; but, he or she may be unsuccessful at finding the income or the personal satisfaction which many seek after early retirement. The result may be a sense of lost purpose or value. For some, it can mean real economic hardship. Creative new living arrangements are becoming available to aging persons, offering varied alternative living possibilities instead of the extremes of managing alone in one's own home or going into a nursing home. However, not all such arrangements are beneficial to the persons they claim to serve. In addition, many cannot afford the care that good retirement living communities offer. Paying for adequate medical and long-term care during the mature years is also a major concern. Elder abuse, like child abuse, seems to be an increasingly visible problem. As life expectancy increases, we face numerous issues about the quality of life for the aging related to competition for society's resources.

Our friends and children, even we ourselves, often fail to understand either the nature or the intensity of our concerns and desires. Both young and old alike may be surprised that we want stimulating work, close personal relations, satisfying sexual relations, and political and economic power. Like younger generations, we usually prefer the company of peers who are active, interesting, and caring. We also appreciate those who no longer behave as others expect them to, but have integrated their life experiences and simply enjoy being themselves. And, we are attracted to those who, like us, are creating new roles for aging persons.

COMPLEMENTARY ROLES

To some teenagers and younger adults in our society, we over 50 have had our chances and are past the age for exploring new opportunities, taking risks, and assuming either authority or responsibility. In their view, we ought to step aside to allow younger people these options. Yet, these ideas are not necessarily irreconcilable with ours, since we may have different priority objectives.

Although our financial concerns often continue, the older we become, the less likely we are to put such things as status, power, recognition, competition, material wealth, and physical attractiveness at the top of our values list. Few of us want to return to the career ladders or organizationally defined roles now held or sought after by younger people. What we do seek is the lifelong opportunity to live with challenge, purpose, and control. We tend to place greater emphasis on life achievement, warm and dependable human relationships, wisdom based on experience, and moral values grounded in religious or cultural traditions.

As women or men who have reached age 50, 60, 70, or 80—leading independent lives, accepting responsibility for our own economic well-being, our own health, and our social relationships—we are not typically persons who need to be told how to live good lives. Admittedly, we face circumstances for which we lack the diverse, attractive examples that were available to us as we approached young or middle adulthood. The roles we have filled as employees, parents, community volunteers, and supportive friends have given us not only accomplishments, but real skills with which to help others as well as ourselves in dealing with the adjustments and transitions typical of adult life.

In addition to this wealth of experience, we often benefit from looking at how a broader group of persons, especially those a few years older than we, grappled with the circumstances of their lives. Some mature women and men make and initiate implementation of their life plans with notable grace. Each of us can recall beautiful persons who turned over their jobs and their community responsibilities, and even adopted new parenting styles, in a manner which enriched the lives of those around them. Of course, we can also recall others who relinquished their authority roles in anguish, prophesying bitterly that things would fall apart without them. Graham Greene said that "In our memories, people we no longer see grow old gracefully." Thankfully, some people we do see also grow old with grace!

LIFE AS DRAMA

"The theater is the house of life."
—ROBERT WILLIAM SERVICE

Imagine your life as a drama played out in a theater—a series of acts and scenes—in which you participate in developing the script as well as playing your role. In most good three-act plays, each of the three acts has numerous scenes, some of them filled with visible, often rapid, action and other scenes which are slower moving and seemingly calm. A few scenes lack much stage movement, but there may be intensive dialogue or a moving soliloquy. Certain scenes may be happy ones, although others will be sad, occasionally even frightening or disturbing.

Using this dramatic analogy, your First Act is composed of the group of scenes in which you played the roles and engaged in the actions of your childhood and student years. Society regarded you as immature and in need of being educated and socialized. Recall the frustrations of trying to become independent within a structure defined by home, school, community, and cultural or religious group? During this First Act, many of us were introduced to strategies for making decisions and were guided by our parents, teachers, counselors, and first employers through a series of steps. We made a series of information-based decisions about education, career, marriage, and location and followed through with plans for action.

Your Second Act began when you entered young adulthood and assumed the various roles of work, family, and community responsibility which normally dominate that period. You probably made decisions about parenthood, owning a home, and establishing an investment or savings account. You were expected to be mature and independent, to earn and save. While some women and men are fortunate enough to feel fulfilled in mid-life, many of us delay the pursuit of certain personal goals until our paid employment ends and our children are grown.

While we generally did not get such specific guidance in the Second Act as we did when we were younger, during our young adult and middle-age years many of us had clear role models for success in family, work, and community life. Recently, both men and women have begun to develop and live according to new patterns based on two-income families or single-parenting. The planning and testing many have done to create these new patterns are similar to that required of us in our later years.

WANTED: EXPERIENCED ACTORS

The Third Act generally begins earlier in many highly developed nations and lasts longer for many people than in prior generations. Planning for the future usually implies projecting from the past. Yet, as I have noted earlier, the huge numbers of mature adults entering this period of our lives have few precedents or conventions to guide us. The average person in past generations died closer to age 50 than 100, and many people were fully employed until shortly before they died. Now, the average life span in both the United States and Great Britain is above age 75 and those over 85 are the fastest growing segment of our population.

In the United States, less than five percent of the elderly are in nursing homes on any given day, although many will spend some time there. Most of us will not have our capacities for independent living limited by chronic illness, poverty, or frailty until a year or two before we die, if at all. We are better educated than the aging in previous generations, with 55 percent of those over 65 in 1989 high school graduates, and a much greater proportion of those approaching 50 college educated. Few of us are wealthy, although only 11 percent were defined as living in poverty according to the 1990 U.S. census.

The more fortunate of us entering our Third Acts have known exceptional people who lived productively and joyfully into their advanced years. Perhaps you have had the privilege of knowing at least one special person severely disabled by heart disease, cancer, limited mobility, or loss of sight or hearing—a man or woman with little hope of getting better. Yet, you felt enriched and joyful after being with that special person. Because of these women and men who had roles in Act III long before us, we are aware of both the possibilities and the perils of growing old.

Still, the daily lives of those special elderly women and men were usually lived out in circumstances quite different from those we are now beginning to experience. In previous generations, elderly people usually lived with or near their children until death, and most spent their final years quietly at home. In some cultures, the elderly were revered for their wisdom and experience. In others, the elderly were sent off to die when they could no longer be productive. None of these conditions is common today in our culture. In many respects, those of us past the age of 50 are writing a new type of life drama.

Among those developing new scripts are the men and women who had expected to have jobs until they are 65, often jobs they have held all of their working years. Now they find themselves being forced to retire from their positions when they are only in their 50s. Wisely, but without preparation for alternatives, many have concluded that "retirement" is not a useful concept or term for describing their new life situation. We are not "retired," but beginning a new phase of purposeful activity. Much more significant than retirement is the concept of planning what to do with the next scenes of our lives.

PREPARING FOR ACT III

"He who is of a calm and happy nature will hardly feel the pressure of Age, but to him who is of an opposite disposition youth and age are equally a burden."

—PLATO

Confronting the opportunity to make something new of yourself can be as frightening as it is exciting. If you view the years after 50 as a time to stay out of the way of the younger generations, you may not enjoy Act III very much. But if you regard your Third Act as an opportunity to act in a number of different scenes offering you various roles and plots, then life takes on new meaning and challenge.

Once you decide to approach life this way, you confront certain tasks and responsibilities related to taking full advantage of your starring dramatic role. You need to determine realistically what your situation is, especially in terms of health, financial status, capacity to deal with change and risk, and the desires and dreams of those with whom you intimately share your life. You also need to examine, perhaps for the first time in years, your values and priorities. What do you care most about? If you cannot do all you would like, what is it most important to do?

Good scripts for your Third Act scene require not only self-understanding and a willingness to accept change, but also accurate information and examples of what men and women experience as they grow older—the challenges and feelings. Research indicates that there are several recurring themes or needs through adult life. Each of these needs should be considered as you plan for new life scenes.

These include not only food and shelter, but also a sense of personal identity, intimacy rather than isolation, a feeling of personal control, opportunities for growth and renewal, adequate fitness and competence for the tasks you undertake, and a feeling of belonging, as opposed to feeling marginal or irrelevant.

Either by design or by accident, we do make choices about our lives. As Harvey Cox has said, "Not to decide is to decide." Based on the above guidelines, which are elaborated more fully through the characters and strategies presented in the following chapters, you can develop your own script for Act III, possibly a broad plan which will answer the questions of what your location and setting will be and how you will pay for this "production." These are all difficult decisions, requiring frequent reconsideration, since none of us knows how long or how expensive our forthcoming scenes will be.

CREATING OUR THIRD ACT SCRIPTS

You will probably develop specific parts of your plan—the scripts for your separate scenes—as you begin to act your part. These detailed plans will be based on the situations and people you encounter and on your resources for dealing with conditions that were carried over from preceding scenes. In other words, your new scenes will depend not only on the typical or unique losses you will inevitably experience, but also on your responses to the opportunities which you recognize and seize.

We star in a series of scenes after age 50, each scene following from the earlier scenes in Act III, and from Acts I and II. Sometimes, the flow from one to the next is almost unnoticed. In others, you will be in a transformed setting, changing your costume, or meeting different characters. In each new scene, you will act out a different scenario or plot. As the main character you will develop and change throughout this process, although the major themes of your life will probably remain the same.

Some people handle these scene changes extremely well, while others either fail to develop their new scripts or do not handle them gracefully. We are most likely to handle new situations well when they result from our own active decisions to make changes. Sometimes we just lose interest or lack the energy to do what we previously did. Most of us have more trouble dealing with changes which are forced on us, either because of our own losses or the wishes of other people, than we do with those we initiate ourselves.

Both my reviews of the research literature and my interviews with aging people indicate that people generally manage the major transitions of their lives most effectively when they know and use planning and decision-making strategies. Regrettably, our personal strategy often is to avoid the subject of aging. It should be no surprise that we feel depressed or out of control when some incident or set of circumstances—in addition to the mirror—forces us to recognize the changes in ourselves. Confronting change is less difficult if we permit ourselves to be aware of the transitions in the lives of others, either by personal acquaintance or through stories. We have so much to learn and so much pleasure to be gained by allowing ourselves to get closer to those in the age groups ahead of us. To dislike old people is to hate yourself, since old is what we are all becoming. As Maurice Chevalier is credited with saying, "Old age isn't too bad when you consider the alternative."

We become discouraged from planning the Third Act of our lives when we realize how often the best of plans have to be revised. Certainly, we have known people who made some key decisions for the later years and then a crisis occurred which made their planned lifestyle impossible. However, the fact that circumstances will change is a reason to plan rather than not to plan. After all, change is a constant in our society and we can consider how to handle it without knowing the specific changes we will encounter.

Some people are "paper planners," while others, probably a large majority, are "head planners." I know men and women who schedule definite times for planning, perhaps New Year's Day, an anniversary, or a religious holiday. I know still more people who are motivated to plan when they hear stories about someone else facing a major change. Then there are the "ostriches," people who keep their heads in the sand and never plan, reacting only when a crisis confronts them directly. Ostriches will have little use for this book.

It is advisable to develop a broad plan for the Third Act of our lives. Both flexibility and specificity are important. Most of us want to leave plenty of room for improvisation, but we all prefer good story lines and well-conceived scripts. We will probably revise our scripts many times. How much easier it is to revise than to do the first draft! Flexibility is a characteristic often thought to be atypical of the aging. It is true that many of us assume the right to state our views and preferences more boldly than in our younger years. After all, one of the benefits of being over 50 is that we can be ourselves. Maybe we are just saving whatever flexibility we can muster for dealing with the numerous transitions we know lie ahead!

DRAMATIC TENSIONS

Life's Third Act may appear to be fraught with dramatic tensions and ambiguities. Is this a tragedy or a comedy? Can change be constant? What is "young old" as opposed to "old old"? Can we plan to be in control when there is a good possibility that for some period of our lives—days, months, or years—we will be dependent on others? How can we as mature persons respect ourselves and our peers in a society which seems eager to push us out of the job market and displays so little respect for its elderly? We probably all know stories of an elderly woman who refused to meet or to live in a retirement community with other women of the same age, saying something like, "I don't want to be with all of those crazy, old ladies."

These apparent contradictions are problematic. My fantasy obituary begins, "She lived for 90 active, joyful, and productive years before dying peacefully in her sleep following a pleasant evening conversing by the fireplace with those she most loved." You may hope for a similar experience, not only for yourself, but also for those you love.

Needless to say, this is not often the way the story ends. For many, there are numerous scenes in the drama of life which are unrehearsed and difficult to play. A disproportionate number of these scenes happen in the Third Act. It is your responses to these conditions which define the play as a tragedy or as a comedy, not the situations themselves.

While we can take some steps to provide for better physical and emotional health in our mature years and can save some portion of what we earn, we cannot expect to control all that happens to us. Still, most of us can be responsible for whether we continue to grow and develop throughout our Third Act, rather than giving up and letting things happen.

It often seems difficult to comprehend change as a constant in our world rather than a crisis. Yet, experience has taught us that throughout history both individuals and societies experience frequent change. The pace of societal change has increased amazingly during our adult lives. Certainly, we are each unique and different from one another. Still, areas of personal change are fairly predictable. Some elderly people do become physically ill, emotionally unpredictable, or mentally incompetent. This is not true for all persons. If such losses do occur, it is generally during the last two years of life or during periods of acute illness.

For most of us, the Third Act will hold 20 to 40 years which can be rich and full. But, those who become dependent on others should have access to the best possible quality of life our society can provide. Everyone has much to gain from this policy. There can be much contagious joy in elderly persons who share their gifts of grace by accepting the caring and sharing of others.

Admittedly, some issues surrounding care for the infirm elderly are public policy issues which we cannot change by ourselves. Still, we cannot deny our individual responsibilities to plan as well as we can for these final scenes. Since some of us will lose the capacity to manage our personal and/or financial affairs, it is critical to our sense of control that we develop and effect clear financial and legal plans covering such contingencies while we are fully capable of doing so.

Each of us will need to be aware of when to withdraw from specific responsibilities. I hope to be sensitive to, and trusting of, the judgments of family, friends, and advisors whether their concerns are explicit or implied. We may need others to help us recognize that the time has come to resign from chairing the church trustees or the local historical society, to give up a driver's license even when the motor vehicle department is willing to re-license us, or to take advantage of community programs designed to assist the elderly to stay in their own homes.

Most of us are doing all we can to stay independent and in good health. Many of us fear loss of our independence more than we do our own deaths. Yet as we reach our 60s, 70s, and 80s, we need to consider how we will handle becoming limited in our capacities and ultimately, how to face our own death—just as many of our ancestors did. Having said that, the emphasis in this book is on continuing to develop new scenes, to make new plans for ourselves, as if the future were largely open-ended. The stories in the chapters which follow demonstrate both the similarities and the differences among the aging. We do not all have the same number of minutes, hours, days, years, or even decades. You and I may have more time on stage than we expect. I, for one, want a Third Act role which permits me to experience innumerable challenging and meaningful scenes. As C.S. Lewis said, "The Future is something which everyone reaches at the rate of sixty minutes an hour, whatever he does, whoever he is."

Productive Scenes or Unresolved Crises

CHAPTER TWO

*"Old age is the most unexpected of all
the things that happen to a man."*

—LEV TROTSKY

APPROACHING NEW SCENES

Let's meet some people in different cycles or stages of mature life. The Endicotts, the Rodriguezes, and the Stines each face critical issues caused by change, issues typical for people between the ages of 50 and 70. Throughout their stories you will see the common themes of people facing challenge and loss, finding new meaning and identity, and struggling to stay in control of their lives. These are serious dramatizations, not melodramas or naturalistic theater. The people portrayed are not on the fringes of society, nor are they women and men who have been either chronically ill or noncontributing members of society. They are typical of the capable persons who live productive lives.

Each has had problems, as ordinary people do, but all of them have managed their own lives without being in a constant state of crisis. Unfortunately, it is not melodrama, but honesty, that forces us to admit that many people have had more social, economic, or health problems than the Endicotts, the Rodriguezes, or the Stines. The challenges such men and women face in aging are even more troubling and difficult to manage.

Now, whether or not they recognize it, each of our actors is approaching a new scene in his or her life's drama with a set of critical decisions to be made. To persons outside their families, the lives of these couples would appear relatively normal, except during certain periods of critical illness. Yet, these "young old" people often feel that things are changing all around and within them. Some of them sense their need to get a new "grip" on life, maybe a new acting coach, but they have few clues about how to do that. For most, some responsibilities from their younger years continue, such as financial support for their children. But they face new tasks and concerns, like caring for infirm parents or spouses. As T.S. Eliot said, "The years between fifty and seventy are the hardest. You are always being asked to do things and yet you are not decrepit enough to turn them down."

Note as you read these profiles that some of the changes in our actors' lives have positive results. There are fresh, often unexpected, sources of joy and productivity for most of these people. The potential for creative action in the next scene often depends on how open the actor is to playing unaccustomed roles. You may want to read each of the brief stories twice, first to see how their experience matches your own or that of people close to you, and then again to identify what specific challenges and decisions each faces now and in the near future.

PROFILE #1

SARAH AND JAMES ENDICOTT

*"The real curse of being old is the ejection
from a citizenship traditionally based on work."*

—Alex Comfort

Sarah, age 50, and James, age 54, have lived in Decatur, Illinois, for 17 years, ever since James became a Ralston Purina department manager. Their three children—Joan, Donald, and Paul—all graduated from public school in Decatur. Now, they either work or attend college at least 50 miles away. Eight years ago, when Joan left for college, Sarah took a job with a real estate firm, where she was promoted to the position of office manager. After their move to Decatur, both Sarah and James became active volunteers, Sarah primarily with activities related to their children's lives and James as a local United Way board member, a role encouraged by his company. In recent years, they gave up the activities they had once been involved in to support their children's interests and now find that they have many fewer obligations.

James became disillusioned with what he regarded as the power struggles among United Way's board members and agencies. He declared that he would never serve on such a community board again. Sarah is, however, quite involved with their local church and currently serves as lay leader. While James sometimes attends worship services, his community interests are primarily in town planning and zoning. He also is an avid golfer, a sport he first started to increase his business contacts, but one he presently enjoys as an escape from work. He says that he can do his worshipping on the golf course by being with nature.

The Endicotts went through a difficult period coinciding with the time when their youngest child, Paul, left for college. For several months James had an affair with a female co-worker, a situation he still isn't quite sure why he allowed to develop. After Sarah learned of the affair through a neighbor's clues, they began seeing a counselor and continued to do so for about a year. Under the counselor's guidance, both James and Sarah recommited themselves to their marriage, but also made decisions to actively pursue some projects individually as well as to spend some planned time together. James has not really found a hobby which interests him, but his work keeps him too busy to worry about initiating a new activity. To her husband, Sarah seems to have become quite independent and self-confident, as James often challenged her to be. Nevertheless, he finds the changes in his wife unsettling.

Since James has become eligible for five weeks of annual vacation time, he and Sarah have taken two long vacations in the past three years, once to Hawaii and another to visit friends in New England and New York. Both as a couple and separately, the Endicotts have developed several circles of friends in Decatur over the years. Recently two couples, who were close friends although a little older than Sarah and James, retired and left Decatur for warmer and, hopefully, less expensive areas of the country. James's older brother had accepted an early retirement offer two years earlier. He and his wife regularly touted the joys and freedom of retirement.

Since their move to Decatur, the Endicotts have lived far from family members other than their children. The three children seem glad to get together for holiday meals, although both Joan and Donald are married and spend holiday time with their in-laws and in their own homes. Not even Paul spends vacations at home anymore, so their visits are brief. Joan is expecting their first grandchild soon, much to Sarah's delight.

Sarah's parents retired to Scottsdale, Arizona, 10 years

ago and are active there, although her Dad no longer seems to enjoy golf because of leg problems. James's father died many years ago in an automobile accident. His mother, 77, moved in with his sister and her husband in Montana after she broke her hip in a fall two years earlier. So far, neither Sarah nor James have been called on to provide direct care or support for relatives, other than their children. However, they have friends who report difficult financial or medical situations involving aging parents.

James is discouraged about his job. He reluctantly concludes that he will never become a division manager and finds that his department will face considerable change in the next year. Just when he is less in agreement than he has ever been with the direction the company is taking and the methods he is expected to use to meet escalating production goals, James is given even higher production targets. There are days when he feels that there is no one around who seems to appreciate all that the department has accomplished under his leadership. The man who hired him for the company was somewhat of a mentor to him in his early years there. They remained friends, and James was deeply saddened by his death the previous year.

When a colleague, who had started with Ralston Purina the same year he did, also died suddenly, James began to wonder how long he could keep up this pace. His own health was good, although his doctor, a golfing partner, advised him at the time of his last physical exam to lose 10 pounds and to reduce his smoking. Sarah experienced health problems a few years before, but hormones and an exercise program seemed to help. In fact, Sarah claims that menopause is the best thing to happen to her in decades, and that she feels more energetic than she has since before her children were born. She occasionally worries about the risk of breast cancer related to using hormones, especially since a close friend recently had breast cancer surgery.

In addition to the fact that James's energy and enthusiasm for new corporate plans and goals are waning, he realizes that some of the new managers are not much older than his own children. When James is invited to attend a company meeting to hear about an early retirement offer, he is startled to be included. He realizes, however, that he is interested in the possibilities. He and Sarah have assumed that James would work until age 65, but the world is changing faster than they expected. Their children are largely self-supporting; the company has a decent pension plan; and their home mortgage is almost paid off. Could he retire at this point, or, at least, before age 65?

James hesitates to tell Sarah about the early retirement offer. His wife has never been happier. She is free of daily parenting tasks, delighted with her leadership role in the church, and enjoys her real estate job. Although Sarah often says she was never much of a student, she talks about preparing for the real estate broker's exam. To James it seems that she is flourishing as she transfers her mothering skills to both her job and the church, where so many depend on her. He wonders how Sarah would respond to the possibility of moving up his retirement date. He is not even sure what he wants to do. There are so many interrelated decisions.

Occasionally they talk of selling their home and moving to a smaller house or another community when James retires. At one time, they even considered buying a cottage on the Lake of the Ozarks and then adding on to it when they retired. The children were teenagers at the time, however, and were not interested in being away from their friends during the summer, so their parents dropped the idea. Now James was glad they had not pursued that plan, as he lost interest in the Ozarks and would not wish to retire there. Still, he does not know where he or Sarah would prefer to live.

Until he has more information about the early retirement program and works with his accountant to project some numbers, he doesn't know whether they can afford to stay in their large family home in Decatur. They count on the increased equity in their home to support their retirement and, of course, would need to sell the house to have access to the money. However, James hasn't wanted to sell before he was 55 because of the tax advantage.

What about their children? How would James's retirement and, possibly, a move away from the area affect them? While the children are all living away from home, Paul still has a year more of college and little chance of a good job for awhile because of the economy. Joan's marriage has been going through a rough period, although her pregnancy apparently has improved the situation. Donald reportedly was very happy with a new wife and a good job, although James believes that the best of jobs, and even marriages, are vulnerable. He and Sarah agree that their children are independent adults. Yet, both are aware that some of their friends' young adult children have returned home to live. Will their children need that type of support?

James finally decides to talk with Sarah while taking her out for dinner. His wife knows him well enough to know that there is some special concern, so she is not completely surprised when he tells her about the early retirement offer.

As James and Sarah consider the possibilities for major changes in their lives, they agree that this is both the "best of times" and the "worst of times"—best because they now have much of what they have had for so long planned and worked toward, and worst because they must begin the difficult work of making specific plans for the indefinite number of mature years of their lives. The first two acts of their lives are ending, and they are planning to enact what Cicero referred to as "Old age: the crown of life, our play's last act."

Key Issues for the Endicotts

In deliberately random fashion, some of the key issues for Sarah and James are listed below. You probably could identify other conditions which also would be regarded as issues for resolution, because you bring your own personal experience to the story. In chapters 5 and 6, these issues and those prompted by the stories to follow will be used as the basis for discussing planning strategies for the mature years:

- James's unexpected push into early retirement;
- James's feeling of having lost colleagues important to his sense of identity;
- Uncertainty about the economic consequences of retirement;
- Contrast between James's dissatisfaction with his life and Sarah's sense of fulfillment;
- Sarah's strong personal ties with local friends of long standing, as well as her continuing church and work relationships;
- Some concerns for their adult children and uncertainty about their own parental roles at this point;
- Unknown potential for future responsibilities for their aging parents;
- Expectations for continuation of reasonably good health; and
- General lack of plans for the future or discussions about new lifestyles and roles they will assume in the distant future.

PROFILE #2

JERRY AND MARIA RODRIGUEZ

> *"Ah, when to the heart of man*
> *Was it ever less than a treason*
> *To go with the drift of things,*
> *To yield with a grace to reason.*
> *And bow and accept the end*
> *Of a love or a season?"*
>
> —ROBERT FROST

Jerry, age 64, and Maria, age 61, grew up in separate neighborhoods in the Bronx, New York. They met in high school and married soon after Maria graduated. Jerry never completed his bachelor's degree at City College, since Anna, their first child, was born within months of Jerry and Maria's marriage, creating new financial demands. In the early years of their marriage, it seemed that every time Maria was ready to find a job, another child was on the way, with Ortiz born two years after Anna, and Juan arriving 18 months later. Their fourth child, Peter, was born 10 years after Juan, an unexpected joy and challenge.

When he left CUNY, Jerry found work as an apprentice plumber. Within two years, he was highly regarded by Fix All Plumbers, Inc., where for 14 years he earned a good salary. Still, as he approached 40, Jerry became frustrated with the limitations of increasing his income as a salaried employee, while his family continued to grow and developed more expensive needs. Jerry decided, with Maria's agreement, that he should start his own plumbing business, Reliant Rodriguez, Inc.

For a few years, their family income was unsteady, but by the time Jerry was 45, he had built a solid business, which also employed their two older children, Anna and Ortiz. Maria helped Jerry in the early years of their business by taking phone calls and doing the billing. After Jerry hired additional plumbers for his firm, they decided to move the business out of their home. At that time, Jerry hired an office manager who took over Maria's duties and some additional tasks. Maria considered taking college courses, but discarded that idea as she became the active, but unpaid, coordinator for volunteers in their area hospital.

Busy with her hospital role, their four children, a series of new grandchildren, and being a companion to Jerry, Maria's life between ages 40 and 60 was almost always full and satisfying. Recently, she has realized she is tiring of the hospital role and finds her children and grandchildren are too busy to spend much time with her. Their business and family activities so fully occupied them all of their adult lives that neither Jerry nor Maria developed many close friends, although they are acquainted with others who are members of their parish.

Like most families, they have had their concerns. Peter, the baby of the family, seems destined for one problem after another. His older sister and brothers feel that Peter is undisciplined and spoiled in comparison with them, but their priest and some of Peter's teachers believe he has either physical or psychological problems which cause his scrapes and his poor grades. Peter eventually graduated from high school, although he still works only part time, and his parents suspect that he is using drugs. Juan enlisted in the Air Force where he served in both Panama and Saudi Arabia. He recently divorced his wife and rarely sees his two children.

Jerry's parents died before he and Maria were married. Her parents returned to San Juan after their youngest child left home. Maria's father died shortly after her parents went to Puerto Rico. For many years, Maria's mother spent each spring in the Bronx with her daughter's family. She is now somewhat confused and feeble and is confined to a nursing home near San Juan. Maria regrets not seeing her mother often, but feels her visits are neither welcome nor remembered. She hopes that her hospital work will somehow help others even though she seems unable to be of much comfort to her own mother. There will soon come a time when Maria will need to return to her childhood home to bury her mother and settle her affairs.

Both Anna and Ortiz continue to work at Reliant Rodriguez. Anna is the office manager and Ortiz a journeyman plumber. Unfortunately, Anna's husband and Ortiz do not get along. This often strains relations between Anna and Ortiz in the business as well as at family gatherings. These tensions concern Jerry, especially since he always intended to turn the business over to his two older children with the understanding that Juan and Peter would also have stock in the corporation.

Jerry and Maria occasionally mention retiring when Jerry reaches age 65. They also talk vaguely of moving to Florida, away from the pressures and winters of New York City. Neither wishes to retire to Puerto Rico, having lived in the States for all of their teenage and adult years. Maria is eager to move to Florida, where she envisions a life of relaxation and friends, with their children and grandchildren visiting during vacations. Given the problems between Anna and Ortiz, Jerry is reluctant to proceed with these plans. He is concerned that the disagreements would cause the loss of good employees and reduce business, affecting both his children's welfare and his own retirement income.

All of this is thrown into new perspective when Jerry is rushed to the hospital early one morning suffering from a heart attack. For days, Jerry and Maria seem unable to get the cardiologist to explain how much damage has occurred. The internist finally explains to them that Jerry should no longer plan to work as a plumber and, in fact, should not plan to return to a full day's work within the next several months, if at all. He indicates that either the stress of physical labor or that of managing the business would be too difficult for his patient's system given the extensive tissue damage.

Maria and Jerry decide to wait a couple of months before making any permanent decisions about the business and their future. During this period, Maria is ill with flu from which she recovers slowly. One morning, Maria looks at herself in the mirror and, for the first time, sees an old woman—slightly overweight, with wrinkled skin and dull eyes. Fortunately, Jerry gradually grows stronger, following a routine of regular rest and a new low-fat diet.

For the first two weeks after his return from the hospital, Jerry talks with his office several times daily and considers having the customer telephones redirected into their home so he can be sure calls are taken promptly and appointments scheduled. Anna and Ortiz, as well as other employees, succeed in convincing him that business is going very well under the regular arrangements. Jerry finally drops the idea and realizes that he thinks less frequently about the office as the days pass.

Jerry becomes interested in using the computer he originally installed at home in order to handle some confidential business records. Since his teenage years, Jerry has remembered and recounted stories of humorous incidents on the job. His fund of stories about skilled laborers and their work often entertained his family and co-workers. Anna, who loves her father's stories, encourages him to write down some of them. Jerry discovers that the computer makes the task easier, since he can easily revise his work. He begins to spend a few hours each day recalling and writing these old stories. Anna's 10-year-old son announces that hearing his grandfather's stories is more fun than watching the programs his parents allow him to watch on TV. Maria enjoys laughing with Jerry and occasionally helps in finding the right way to tell part of a story.

Since Maria stays home more than in the past in order to be with Jerry, she also has opportunities to share coffee with Jolene, a new neighbor who does a number of different crafts. It has been many years since Maria has done any creative work of this type. When Jolene asks her to help by making some dolls for the hospital's craft fair, Maria discovers that she not only enjoys the work but is good at it. Might this be a better way for her to support the hospital than serving as the volunteer coordinator? Maria decides to phase out of her position at the hospital.

For several months, Jerry and Maria spend more time at home than either have in years. Gradually they settle into a routine which includes daily walking, relaxed meals, and individual project work—writing stories for Jerry and crafts for Maria. At first, it takes Maria considerable time to plan and prepare the low-fat diet prescribed for Jerry, but she finds it easier as she becomes familiar with the different buying and cooking habits required. They each spend some time keeping in touch with their past responsibilities, the plumbing business for Jerry, and the hospital volunteer association for Maria. Although neither mentions the matter, both feel that it is important to set a schedule which includes some time spent apart from each other daily.

Occasionally, they invite another couple or two from their parish to share one of Maria's new recipes, a type of social life that they had often talked about, but for which they had previously found little time. Both are privately pleased that their sexual relations have become as pleasurable as they were in their young adult years, although they have intercourse much less frequently than when they were young. Once in a while, either Maria or Jerry mentions that they don't seem to be doing anything much of real value. Jerry comments to his son that he feels invisible to the rest of the world now that he is not active in the business. Yet, Anna tells her mother that she has never seen her parents so content.

When Jerry and Maria agree that the time has come to talk about the business and where they will live in the next stage of their lives, they are glad they have waited awhile after Jerry's hospitalization to do so. A year ago, the Rodriguezes thought of themselves as middle-aged. Now, there is a new, but rather unclear, sense of reality about themselves. They find the decisions they face full of both possibility and regret, for they are becoming aware that they will have to give up some of what they value in order to satisfy their new interests and needs.

Key Issues for the Rodriguezes

The Rodriguezes face a different set of issues from the Endicotts. For example, Jerry has more control over his actual retirement decision than did James because he owns the business; however, his heart attack reduces the possibilities for him in ways that James has not experienced. Because the Rodriguezes are older than the Endicotts, they have fewer unknown circumstances related to their children and aging parents. In their early 60s, Jerry and Maria face the following issues. Again, you will see additional issues because of your own life experience:

- Both major and minor physical changes;
- Unresolved situations with young adult children and an aging parent;
- Children and growing grandchildren busy with their own activities;
- Loss of recognized work roles and tasks for both Maria and Jerry;
- Decisions about where to live in retirement;
- Financial, legal, and operational questions about transferring the family business;

- Changing interpersonal relationships within both family and community;
- Sense of being out of the mainstream of life;
- Development of new interests, activities, and pleasures; and
- Timing decisions for business and personal changes.

PROFILE #3

SYBIL AND LARRY STINE

*"With age, we become responsible for what's in our heads—
the character of the memories there, the music we are
familiar with, the storehouse of books we have read,
the people whom we can call, the scenery we know
and love. Our memories become our dreams."*

—EDWARD HOAGLAND

Sybil, age 70, and Larry, age 73, happily sold their home in Cleveland Heights, Ohio, to live in Coral Gables, Florida, when Larry retired from the tire business seven years before. They decided to live an active and simplified life playing tennis and enjoying Florida's warm weather. Much of their formal furniture they gave to their sons, Jake and Barry. One of their daughters-in-law did a great deal of entertaining and was pleased to take most of Sybil's serving dishes and table linens. She gave her fur to the other daughter-in-law and donated their winter clothes to a Jewish charity. Sybil also insisted that "the boys" take all of their childhood mementos and most of the photo albums and movies accumulated over the years, keeping only a few special ones. It felt good to "lighten their load."

They made a profit on the increase in value of their home and projected that they could live very well throughout the remainder of their lives and still leave a respectable inheritance to their sons. The Stines had vacationed in the Miami area for a number of years and were well acquainted there through both their tennis club and their synagogue. In the early years of retirement, their lives were filled with tennis matches, cocktail parties, dinners out, and visits from their two sons and their young families. Friends from Cleveland Heights often came to visit as well, seeming to envy the lifestyle Sybil and Larry established.

Larry was a naval officer in World War II and became reacquainted with some friends from those days who also retired to Florida. Sybil claimed her husband's navy buddies forgot their ages and lived in the past, but Larry enjoyed the camaraderie. He also spent several hours each week managing his stock investments, a task previously performed by his broker. Sybil had managed their household accounts all of their married lives, but she turned these over to Larry when he retired, figuring he needed to be busy.

Sybil truly missed her Cleveland Heights friends and their large home and garden; however, she enjoyed their relaxed life and the warm climate, certainly better for her arthritis than the cold winters of Cleveland. Then just before her 69th birthday, Sybil suffered a stroke which paralyzed the left side of her body. Hospitalization for Sybil meant a difficult 10-day period for Larry as well. For two or three days, he was quite fearful of losing her and could see her for only five minutes each of the several hours that she was in intensive care. When she was moved to a double hospital room, there seemed to be an ever-changing group of hospital personnel whose names and functions he could seldom get straight. In spite of the many staff, there were often times when no one seemed to be available to assist Sybil with eating or using the bedpan.

More than once, Larry arrived back in Sybil's room after a trip home or a meal in the hospital's cafeteria to discover that an attendant, after changing the bed linens, had failed to return the nurse call button to a location which Sybil could reach. Just when they seemed to be developing a predictable routine, Sybil got a new roommate, a woman whose numerous family and friends appeared to visit in noisy crowds, all speaking Spanish. It was very important to Sybil that she reconstruct mentally what had happened to her and where she had been in the preceding days. She was sure she had had several blood transfusions, but seemed unable to confirm that. Larry was able to help her with many of the details, but he did not find a chance to ask her physician or the head nurse, and no one else seemed to be permitted to disclose such details.

After a week, the nurse told them that the doctor said Sybil could soon return home. But, the day before she was to leave, a urinary tract infection was diagnosed. They learned that this is not unusual in cases where a catheter is used for an extended period of time because of the patient's immobility. Still, it required more days in the hospital and was cause for concern. Fortunately, during this period physical therapists taught Sybil how to use a motorized wheelchair. Finally, with instructions about assisting Sybil to and from the wheelchair, a physician's appointment scheduled a few weeks later, and an invitation to call if there were problems, Larry took Sybil home to their condo. Both Sybil and Larry knew that they were returning to a different life.

Larry had called both Jake and Barry shortly after Sybil's stroke. Their sons were worried and wanted to know what they could do. Larry told them not to come, that he would keep in touch with them about their mother's progress. He talked with each of them regularly during their mother's hospitalization; however, since their jobs and personal lives were complicated right now, he did not feel that he could ask them to come. Instead, he reported that he was managing well and that they both looked forward to visits from them when they could arrange it.

When they first returned home, Sybil felt Larry hovering over her. She was frustrated by her limitations and was often irritable. Eventually, she suggested that Larry buy a small dinner bell and a portable telephone so she could call him. After her "command control station" was set up, she told him to either sit down in another room or go out and do something—like play tennis at the club. Larry tried to resume a more normal pace, but his life and concerns had been irrevocably changed too. After seeing the physician several times and going to physical therapy, they realized that Sybil would probably be confined to a wheelchair, although her upper body mobility seemed to be improving. With equal amounts of therapy and determination, Sybil learned to use a motorized wheelchair skillfully, to cook modest meals, and to care for herself, primarily using her right arm and hand. Since she could no longer climb the stairs of their condominium, they arranged to move the upstairs bedroom furniture to the downstairs den. They also had their kitchen remodeled so that Sybil could reach the sink, stove, and refrigerator from her wheelchair.

In some ways, the greatest loss for Sybil seemed to be her self-confidence. As a result of the stroke, the left side of her face was slightly distorted. While others hardly noticed the change, Sybil herself was very self-conscious about her appearance and limited capacities and became reserved and withdrawn from all except a few of their friends. They seldom went out to eat anymore, since Sybil said that she could not be sure of wheelchair accessibility and it was such a project to get ready to go. Larry sensed that it was her self-consciousness about her appearance that really prevented their going.

Larry was reluctant to resume an active tennis and social schedule alone. Consequently, the Stines refused most invitations and seldom invited others to visit. After awhile, few people invited them, although some telephoned occasionally to see how they were. Larry spent much of his time reading financial magazines and, increasingly, took on managing their household, formerly Sybil's role. He made a few false starts at being helpful, the major example being his attempt to surprise Sybil by fixing some microwave popcorn. Only when the flames began did Larry learn that he should have removed the cellophane wrapping from the package. After the mess was cleaned up, they enjoyed a good laugh and Larry agreed that he would ask Sybil's advice prior to trying something new in the kitchen.

Sybil had been an active reader of fiction, but now complained that the books and magazines she was given by friends were "not her type" and that she had read everything else in the house. Larry seemed unable to figure out what her "type" was, and was not much help in selecting reading materials. They watched television together each morning and evening and began to follow a number of programs regularly. Since they didn't always agree on which programs to watch, occasionally Larry watched his programs in the upstairs bedroom he now used as a den. Sybil commented more than once that Larry turned the TV volume so high that she thought he was losing his hearing, a subject he refused to discuss.

They talked from time to time about moving to a place all on one level, and even dreamed about the possibilities of a small garden once again. Sybil and Larry seemed happiest when they shared memories of their years in Cleveland and their first years in Florida when the children and grandchildren visited often. Their sons gave them a fine entertainment unit and a complete CD player after their move to Coral Gables. But they seldom played the CD, although they both enjoyed music and were regular in their attendance at musical events in the Cleveland area. Larry especially enjoyed musical theater, while Sybil loved light opera. By chance, Larry found that a golfing friend had an extensive CD collection, so he arranged to borrow some of the music they liked. Sybil seemed invigorated and cheered by the music, and they began to play tapes regularly during dinner and often on into the evenings when they didn't watch television.

Larry did not mention his concerns to Sybil, but their on-going bills related to her illness, as well as reduced earnings on their investments, were making it difficult to pay the escalating membership and maintenance fees for the condo from their income. Yet he was reluctant to draw down the principal of their assets at this point in their lives. Not only was the condo expensive, but they were paying for recreation privileges and for upper floor household space they could no longer fully use. He wasn't at all sure how Sybil would deal with the knowledge of their financial situation or the possibility of a move to another location. Although his wife's stroke hadn't affected her mental capacities, Larry thought she became emotional and easily upset by even minor problems. Larry readily understood that Sybil's physical limitations and her occasional pain accounted for her responses. He himself often felt rather depressed about the changes in their situation. Larry also decided not to mention that his physician had diagnosed an enlarged prostate; however, Sybil certainly was aware of his increased frequency and urgency to urinate and sensed he had a problem that would surely require medical attention.

In addition to their reduced social activity in Coral Gables, there were fewer visits from Cleveland-area friends and from their children. Their older son, Jake, now 46, had taken a position in Los Angeles, where his wife was also employed. Jake's two children were teenagers and had very active school and community schedules. Their younger son, Barry, 44, had just ended a prolonged divorce process and started a new marketing firm in Boston. He occasionally came to Miami on business, but seemed to have time for little more than a quick phone call now and then. Although Sybil was very fond of Barry's ex-wife and doted on their grandchildren, neither she nor Larry had seen Barry's three children or his ex-wife for three years. Before Sybil's stroke, they had discussed offering to fly the children to Miami for a vacation, but that subject hadn't been discussed recently. Since they had not seen Barry's children for some time, they were not sure that the children would want to come. After Sybil's illness, she and Larry each wondered privately how they would handle it if their active, young grandchildren did visit.

Sybil eventually broke their self-imposed silence by suggesting that she and Larry talk about what they should do over the next several years. She realized that her illness had put additional responsibilities on Larry. In addition, Jake had pointed out to them in a recent telephone conversation that their current living and financial management arrangements were totally dependent on Larry's continuing good health. Jake had really irritated Larry by saying that, at age 73, one shouldn't count on being both physically and mentally independent for too many more years. While Larry was furious and accused Jake of saying he was incompetent, the conversation had set Sybil to thinking and opened the door for their next steps. Given Sybil's physical condition combined with Larry's lifelong independence and his own concerns for their financial situation and his own health, the discussion and resulting changes were bound to be both stressful and necessary.

Key Issues for the Stines

Sybil's stroke caused a sudden, dramatic, and permanent change in lifestyle for the Stines. Some of the other key issues are as follows:

- Distance from long-time friends and family;
- Apparent lack of a support group in Coral Gables;
- Loss of independence for Sybil because of her paralysis;
- Changes in emotional stability and confidence for Sybil;
- Alteration in Sybil's appearance;
- Shift of household responsibilities from Sybil to Larry;
- Physical and emotional distance of the sons in relation to their parents' altered situation;
- Poor or no communication by Larry about both their financial situation and his own health;
- Renewed pleasures in music and gardening;
- Loss of previously enjoyed activities for both; and
- Lack of any script for living beyond the time when both were independent physically and mentally.

Role Changes Under Pressure

CHAPTER THREE

"You don't change when you grow old.
You remain just the same. But everything else
changes. Your home. Your friends. Your city.
The things you are used to just disappear,
one by one. And you are left alone."

—GREGORY CLARK

ROLES FOR THE SEVENTIES

In chapter 2, we met three couples between the ages of 50 and 70 and became acquainted with the changes they are facing. Their issues involve retirement, sudden and life-threatening declines in health, decisions about moving, as well as the interactions between them and their close relatives and friends related to these issues. In this chapter, we meet Bessie Smith and Olivia and John Wilson, who are either approaching or past age 70 when we first meet them.

Having lived through some of the early scenes of the Third Acts of their lives, they are experiencing additional losses and concerns. Both chronic and acute physical ailments and reduced energy become significant issues for these people, as they do for many by the mid-seventies. Realistically understanding the changes and graciously accepting their conditions without giving up may become challenging tasks. Communicating with family members and getting desired support from them without losing our own control can be difficult.

Like these representative characters, some of us develop new understandings and insights during the process of facing the challenges of the 70s. Others regard some of these scenes of their lives as being without hope or joy. Their sense of loss is so great that it masks the new opportunities or insights which might enable them to balance the losses. The people in this chapter are nearing the close of scenes which take place well into the Third Act of their lives and have urgent needs to plan for the next scene as they approach their 80s.

PROFILE #4

BESSIE SMITH

"Life for a year, a month, a day or an hour is still a gift."

—HUGH MACLENNON

Bessie Smith, age 77, was born and raised on the South Side of Chicago. Bessie married Robert, who was four years older, when she was seventeen. They soon moved to Pontiac, Illinois, where Robert found a job as a prison guard. Bessie never graduated from high school, and Robert was 35 years old before he got his GED certificate. They both worked steadily after they reached sixteen. Their marriage was strong, although both wished they had completed high school and gotten either college or technical school training before they married. Based on their own experiences, the Smiths were determined that all four of their children—Jenny, Kevin, Joe, and Lavonna—graduate from high school. In addition, Bessie and Robert promised to help any of their children who did well in high school and wanted to go on to college.

Tragically, Robert was killed in a prison riot when he was 42. Bessie was only 38, and their children were still teenagers or somewhat dependent young adults. Being a single parent and working full time was very difficult for Bessie. The boys especially seemed to miss their father's discipline as well as his income. Jenny had an abortion before her mother even realized that her eldest child was sexually active. During his teenage years, Kevin was often beaten by gang members, who justified their actions by calling him a fag. Joe's friends seemed to stay out of trouble, but they were not much interested in high school or the possibility of college. Lavonna, the youngest, seemed to do well in school and had friends, although Bessie tired of her daughter's concerns with her hair and her clothes.

These early years after her husband's death were lonely and tough. When she looked back, it seemed to Bessie that only her belief in Christ, the support of her church friends, and her usual sense of humor pulled them through.

After her husband's death, Bessie realized that it was up to her to support herself and help Jenny and Kevin finish college, since Robert Smith left only a small life insurance policy and an equal amount of accident insurance. She left her part-time job in Pontiac and drove 30 miles each way to a new position as a file clerk in the auto claims department of State Farm Insurance Company. Over time, Bessie learned how to process claims and handle both policy holder and agent concerns over the telephone.

Either because Bessie lacked the formal education required or because she was black, she was never sent out in the field and was not given either the title or pay of those who did work similar to hers. Still, she enjoyed the work and the contacts with others in the insurance office which provided both meaning and a dependable rhythm to her days. As her children became adults, Bessie's nights were often lonely, except for those evenings she could escape her housework and go to church meetings.

At age 65, Bessie was required to retire from State Farm. She continued to live in Pontiac on her small, fixed pension supplemented by social security, with major medical benefits from her former employer. Three of the Smith children had married and moved some distance away before Bessie retired. They visited when they could; however, after Bessie's grandchildren became teenagers, with their own jobs and friends, their visits were infrequent.

Robert's and Bessie's younger son, Kevin, never married and continued to live in Pontiac with his mother. Kevin graduated from college and was employed as a designer for a small advertising firm in a nearby community. Although he was out much of the time it was a pleasure to have him share dinner with her some evenings. Bessie also appreciated her son's capable way of keeping household equipment and her car in good repair. She worried all of her son's life about his frailty and his frequent ailments and was grateful to have him close by so she could care for him.

After her retirement, Bessie finally had time to be active in both her church choir and a community chorus. She took training and became a volunteer for the local hospice, where she spent three afternoons each week with dying persons or their family members. Her third retirement project was "fixing up" her home like she had always wanted to. How she wished that her husband and children could be around now that she finally had things done right!

Bessie's biggest project was that of unofficial coordinator for the human needs within her local church. Either Pastor Brown or a member of the congregation would call Bessie when someone was dying, was ill, or felt in need of support.

Bessie enlisted others to respond whenever she could. Yet, it was often Bessie who took a casserole and sat with an ill or troubled person when she learned that a family or individual needed support, as she herself had in the early months and years after her husband's death.

It irritated Bessie to find that she required a bit more rest during the daytime than she had during her working years. She attributed her declining energy to the fact she didn't sleep well at night. Increasingly, she had to get up three or four times nightly to urinate and then had trouble getting back to sleep. When she told her doctor of this condition, he said not to worry, that it was normal to sleep less soundly in later years. That advice did not solve the problem, but Bessie worried less about it. Generally, Bessie's many interests and her determination to be active and to help others, as they had helped her after her husband's death, kept her active and happy into her seventy-fifth year.

In recent years, some friends her age seemed to enjoy less and less about their lives. Bessie could certainly understand their depression or complaints when facing the death of a spouse or suffering severe health problems. She also sympathized with those whose relationships with their children and grandchildren were strained or nonexistent. In addition, she lived close enough to the edge of her own financial resources to know why some older friends seemed to speak of nothing other than their medical expenses, food bills, and taxes. It was sad to attend a number of funerals these days, but Bessie was grateful to have lived in Pontiac for most of her adult life and to have shared in the life cycles of many friends. Celebrating these lives through the music of her choir was to Bessie a joyful and fitting end, one she hoped for herself, when the time came.

The winter she was 77, Bessie stumbled and fell one night as she returned home from sitting with her long-time friend, Julia, now dying of inoperable cancer. Fortunately, she had fallen in the house rather than outside. However, she was unable to get up because of intense pain and weakness in her right side. By morning, she struggled to the telephone from which she called Pastor Brown, who arranged for an ambulance and called Kevin at work to alert him of his mother's fall. He met her at the hospital and helped with the admission process. Bessie's doctor contacted a surgeon who operated the next day to set her broken hip.

She went home after a week, returning regularly for therapy and using a walker at home. With her usual enthusiasm for life, Bessie kept in active touch with church and community friends by telephone or through their visits to her home. It seemed odd for Bessie to be receiving the visits, casseroles, flowers, and cards, given her usual role of assisting others.

After Bessie's hip surgery, her three children who were living away from Pontiac tried to call more often than they had before. All four Smith children were now past 50 themselves, some with difficult health or financial problems. Jenny, a long-time smoker, was forced to retire early from her secretarial job in Los Angeles because of emphysema. She found it physically difficult and too expensive to take the long trip back to Illinois. Joe was a foreman at the Honda plant in Maryville, Ohio. It was a good job, but the pressure for job performance kept him from taking more than a weekend off. Besides, his wife was chronically ill and needed his care every evening and weekend after she returned from the adult day care facility. Lavonna had purchased her own beauty shop in Kansas City, but did not yet have confidence that other operators could keep the business going if she was gone for long.

Kevin continued to be both Bessie's major helper and her greatest concern. His infections had become more frequent, and he missed work often. Bessie suspected AIDS, but had not confronted her son with her suspicions, almost afraid that he would tell her what she dreaded to hear. She long ago concluded that Kevin was homosexual, although she had never been aware that he had intimate relationships with other men. Friends in her church and community were not very tolerant of such behavior, so it was difficult for her to share her fears. What would happen if Kevin should become even more ill or, worse, die? Perhaps she had depended on her son for both help and companionship more than was good for either of them.

Sadly, Bessie's friend Julia died two months after her fall; however, Bessie was glad that she could attend the funeral and even sing with the choir. After the funeral, she decided that it was time to shake off her own worries by getting back into her former activities.

A week or so later, Pastor Brown came to call. Bessie assumed he planned to discuss the use of the donations at Julia's funeral, the choir, or the arrangements for assisting several congregational members who were ill. She was startled when he said, "Bessie, some of us believe that you have been trying to do too much for a woman of your age. I have recommended to the church board that they name Ann Jones, whose youngest child graduates from high school this spring, to a new staff position as coordinator of congregational needs. Ann can handle the many telephone calls and personal services which you have provided for so long. We are very grateful to you, but you surely deserve a rest." Sensing Bessie's concern, Pastor Brown reminded her that she did not need to work to earn God's love, quoting Ephesians, "By grace you have been saved through faith; and this is not your own doing, it is the gift of God."

Pastor Brown's call, combined with nagging concerns for her own health and that of Kevin and her awareness of the increasing difficulties of many older friends, nudged Bessie into some serious thinking. She hated to give up her role in the church, although she felt some relief that the urgent needs of people she so loved were being recognized by others. Perhaps it was time for her to receive this change by saying "thank you" to God and to those who would fill her active roles. Bessie knew that she could still extend kindness and joy to others, even if less dramatically.

She admitted to herself that she had put off decisions about the next period of her life. Although none of her children expressed concern about their mother's abilities to live independently, Bessie realized that she probably would become dependent on others at some point in the future. Within a few weeks, she began to accept the fact that some plans had to be made. Bessie did what she had done at other critical points in her 77 years—she turned to God in prayer and asked for guidance in dealing with her life.

Next, she decided to talk with friends and with Pastor Brown about what she should do, now that she was free of some of her earlier responsibilities. Normally not one to make lists, Bessie also decided that this time she should write down some ideas and, then, write to each of her distant children and talk directly with Kevin to ask for their reactions to her plans. Of course, it would be best to get the whole family together. Wouldn't it be wonderful if they all came home for the Fourth of July celebration—like they used to! Maybe some of her 11 grandchildren and 25 great-grandchildren could come too. With renewed energy and enthusiasm, Bessie started a campaign to make that happen. Summer could be a new beginning for this aging lady!

Key Issues for Bessie Smith

At age 77, Bessie Smith has never had the financial resources of some of the people we met earlier. She faced significant loss early with the death of her husband, but since then has stayed very much in control of her life and has been active and happy. Now, much of that happiness and activity seems threatened.

Some of the main conditions and issues are:
- Loss of her informal title as needs coordinator for her church;
- Suspicions about Kevin's health;
- Some concerns for decline in her own health and related capacity for future independence (e.g., hip fracture and frequency of urination);
- Continuing loss of friends to death or debilitating illness;
- Geographical and possible emotional distance from three of her adult children;
- Probable financial limitations on future housing and health care choices;
- Persistence of Bessie's positive, but realistic attitude toward life;
- Strong religious faith; and
- Deep roots in the church and local community.

PROFILE #5

OLIVIA AND JOHN WILSON

"As you grow older, you realize that the only things which are a matter of life and death are life and death."

—RICHARD J. NEEDHAM

As Olivia Wilson looked back on her life, both alone and with her husband, John, she realized that they either lived in or traveled to more places than either of them even knew existed when they first met at Allegheny College. John finished medical school at Columbia three years after they married 55 years ago. Although some of his medical school colleagues were drafted to serve in World War II, either John's specialty or his draft number always kept him from being called into the armed services. Immediately after completing medical school, he took a residency in Los Angeles and then another in pediatric oncology in Chicago. By the time John and Olivia settled in Philadelphia, where John established his practice, the Wilsons had three beautiful children—Jamie, Carol, and Ken.

During the residency periods and in the early years of John's private practice, Olivia tried doing some substitute teaching to improve the family's finances. She finally concluded that her outside work was incompatible with raising young children and never applied for teaching certification in Pennsylvania. Before John was 39 and Oliva 37, they improved their financial position enough to build a large home in an affluent, new suburb. John's hours were long and unpredictable, so it was Olivia who supported the children's activities and helped them with their schoolwork.

While there were many children in their neighborhood, most were enrolled in special lessons, active in competitive sports and after-school clubs. When the children were young, Olivia found herself arranging for playgroups, and later it was parties, games, and trips to Philadelphia that required mothers to drive and supervise. As the children grew older, an increasing number of their friends' mothers worked away from home, leaving only a few mothers to carry the burden of transporting and being available to neighborhood teenagers. Olivia tried to limit her own activities to the time when the children were in school, although she did play golf and tennis with friends during the summers. It was not quite the life Olivia envisioned when she studied literature at Allegheny; however, she was generally glad that John's income allowed her to be home for both him and the children.

John had little interest in financial management, and Olivia often urged him to employ a more experienced office manager for his growing practice—but she had little success. John devoted whatever family time he could to their children and left the home management to his wife. The Wilson children experienced the usual childhood accidents and illnesses, but seemed basically healthy and happy.

All three children did well in school, but they were especially proud when the oldest, Jamie, was named valedictorian of his class and accepted at Yale. Carol starred during her senior year in high school in several dramatic productions. That was the end of her stage career, since she fell in love her first year in college, got married and left school after completing her second year. Ken was the family and class clown, keeping them all wondering when he would ever get serious about his studies and his life.

As the children began to leave home for college, their first jobs, and marriage, Olivia became more involved in the area YWCA. She not only served as its president, but was also on several regional and national committees. She continued to enjoy her neighborhood friends, with whom she shared coffee at least monthly. Still, she realized that the group was changing. Some couples retired, divorced and/or moved away. Even more women seemed to be working outside of their homes, and younger people with diverse racial and ethnic backgrounds were moving into the area. Olivia thought of herself as open-minded; still, she occasionally felt like a stranger in the very neighborhood which she and John had helped to establish.

As the years passed, John's practice continued to expand to the point where he seemed to be on call most of the time. He had a difficult time getting regular exercise, except for a weekly game of tennis. Olivia became concerned that John was gaining considerable weight, but her husband said that he, not she, was the physician and would decide when his weight was becoming a problem. Never a manager or interested in building a business, he had to be persuaded by Olivia and their son Jamie to bring a younger pediatrician into his practice to share the load. Eventually, two others joined the professional staff, requiring additional examination space and more clerical staff. John commented more than once that this group practice felt too scheduled and pressured for his type of medicine.

John had a number of close friends within the medical profession; however, he seemed not to trust lawyers, brokers, and bankers, and turned to David Archer, his accountant, only to do his taxes for his professional practice and the family. Each April at tax time, David raised a number of questions about how John was handling his money, his insurance, and his property and urged him to develop an estate plan; however, Archer was very careful to indicate that he, of course, was not a broker or an attorney and that he did not give advice. Once the taxes were signed and sent off, John was happy to get back to medicine and ignored most of what David had said.

When John reached age 65 and Oliva age 63, they finally agreed to talk about retirement. As a result, they decided that John would sell his interest in the medical practice and would gradually turn his patients over to other pediatricians during the next year. They would also sell their home in Pennsylvania. Then, they would build a new home in a beautiful area in North Carolina, where they had vacationed briefly a few times. Fortunately, John found his partners eager to buy his interest in the professional practice. His feelings were mixed when he realized that much of its value was in his own reputation, and that his share of the practice was of less monetary value than he expected.

Since they had owned their home for many years, it had appreciated considerably in value. The Wilsons made expensive improvements to their home, first as their children grew, and later to suit their own taste. They found that the uncertain economy in 1980 coupled with high mortgage interest rates made it difficult to find a qualified buyer. Younger couples were not prepared to pay for many of the improvements and luxury features which had been added. The result was that they were delayed in selling their home well beyond the time when they started building in North Carolina and, eventually, agreed to a price $200,000 below what they had projected in their retirement planning.

By the time they completed the transfers of the practice and their home and bade farewell to long-time friends and associates in the Philadelphia area, they were exhausted. Olivia attended a seminar for wives whose husbands were retiring and did some recommended reading about the changes couples face when they retire. She also knew that leaving familiar people and surroundings and going into a new community was usually stressful. John, as a physician, had a professional understanding of how changes affected people; however, he seemed able to apply these concepts only to his patients and not to himself or his own family.

As they drove to North Carolina in June to meet the movers in their not-quite-finished new home, Olivia tried to talk with John about the challenges they faced in making these changes. She felt sad and lonely already at leaving her friends behind. On the other hand, she was overjoyed at having more time with her husband and looked forward to the new people they would meet. John did not want to discuss his feelings, although he too seemed depressed and admitted that he was tired. Olivia gave up trying to talk about challenges and tried to emphasize the relaxation and pleasure she hoped were ahead for them.

They both enjoyed the views from their hilltop home, which was completely finished after three months of additional work. The Wilsons' home was located in a community whose residents were invited to join an exclusive local tennis club. Their club offered a swimming pool, a restaurant, and contract bridge groups. John was quickly able to find tennis matches and played at least three times each week. Olivia developed a bad knee the prior summer and had consequently given up tennis. She found that to get acquainted she would have to do something scheduled, so she signed up for bridge. On some days, she felt rather like her children must have when they went from one lesson or scheduled play activity to another!

John and Olivia enjoyed a regular cocktail hour, either with new friends in their home or at the club, or just between the two of them. After John's professional work and Olivia's roles as mother and community leader, their lives occasionally seemed rather empty and without meaning. Still, they tried to emphasize the benefits of being together more and living at a more relaxed pace.

Olivia missed her friends and her family. She invited their children and their families to come down for Christmas. But, their middle-aged children's and teenage grandchildren's schedules were too full at that time of year, it seemed, and none of the families could come. Another year, they promised they would all try to come for a big Christmas celebration. Both John and Olivia were glad that their children kept in touch by telephone and promised to visit when they could. Numerous friends who either still lived in Pennsylvania or had retired to Florida said they would visit. By the end of the year, they had only one set of visitors, so they decided to expand their circle of friends.

One warm afternoon in late January, Olivia took a telephone call from the director of their club. John had collapsed on the tennis court and was taken to the nearest hospital by ambulance. She drove the 10 miles to the hospital by herself and was told that John had suffered a severe heart attack. His condition was described as critical, and it was too soon to give any prognosis for the future. John was in the intensive care unit for three days before he was moved to a private room in the cardiac rehabilitation area. There, he continued to be monitored electronically and was not permitted to get out of bed for several days.

Their older son, Jamie, and their daughter, Carol, each flew down for a few days to be with Olivia and John during the hospitalization period.

Olivia and her daughter were quite concerned that John seemed so discouraged. He talked of not being needed and of being a burden to others. He seemed to believe that he would never again be able to do the things he liked to do, although no one had much success in getting him to describe what activities were most important to him other than tennis.

While the family knew that there had been considerable initial tissue damage, no one would know for several weeks how active John could be in the future. John's physical recovery was good enough that, almost two weeks after his heart attack, he went home. He was released from the hospital with advice to "take it easy" and reduce the calories and fat in his diet, at least for awhile. An appointment was scheduled with the cardiologist's office for a checkup in four weeks, and he was directed to call his internist if he had problems or concerns in the meantime. Since John himself was medically trained, he asked few questions and prevailed on family members not to do so.

Hospital staff helped Olivia load John and his personal supplies into their car. She drove home hoping that John would begin to feel more cheerful and optimistic once he was in their own place. Both Jamie and Carol returned to their homes, where they each seemed to be dealing either with problems related to their in-laws or their own children. Jamie had called the Wilsons' younger son, Ken, in Japan the day after their father's heart attack. It was unlikely that he would return to the States, since the family clown now had a very demanding corporate job in Osaka where his wife and children also lived.

John was glad to be back in their new home again, but talked mostly of the pleasures and activities of their former life and work in Philadelphia. Neither John nor Olivia had had much opportunity to make many friends in North Carolina. Those John did enjoy he knew primarily as tennis players. Friends from Pennsylvania and family members called often in the first few weeks after John became ill. People they had met at the club stopped in several times with flowers, a book, or food—mostly delicacies John probably should not eat. Olivia arranged to have a woman come in for a half day each week to clean. That became a good time for her to get her hair done and pick up some groceries. John was taking care of his personal needs himself, even fixing himself a snack when he was hungry. Still, Olivia felt she should be with him most of the time to assist him and to keep him company.

Four weeks later, the cardiologist gave John a series of tests and told him that they would wait for more healing before they gave him a stress test. Both John and Olivia were hoping to be told that John could expect to resume his active life within a few months as long as he was careful about stress and kept his weight down. When John persisted in his efforts to get a specific prognosis, the cardiologist suggested he make an appointment to see his internist soon and that they make some projections about recovery then. Within a week, Olivia and John talked with the internist; however, the results were not encouraging. He advised John not even to think of tennis for some time, especially since John was so competitive. He suggested that, instead, he take up regular walking, not jogging, and that he find some hobby that interested him.

Olivia began a regular walking routine, but was seldom able to coax John to join her. During the next several months, Olivia, with suggestions from her sons and daughter, tried to introduce John to a variety of possible hobbies—stamp collecting, wood carving, painting, and so on. Nothing really challenged John like his medical practice or tennis matches had. They knew some men who became very active in managing their investments at this stage of their lives. That was hardly appealing to John, who had turned this task entirely over to his broker with directions to make money and arrange for payment of income of the amount they had decided they would need annually. Even reading about investments failed to interest John.

Watching professional tennis and football on television seemed to be the only activity which John regularly enjoyed, so he and Olivia did a great deal of that. They ate dinner at the tennis club a few times, but John complained of the food and the service, both of which he had thought satisfactory before his illness. After a few months, they stopped going. John's broker called every few weeks with ideas about new investments. It seemed to Olivia that their financial arrangements ought to be more settled than they were, but John always told the broker to make whatever changes he thought best.

Olivia tried for the second time to get family members down for Christmas, but without success. When the children called, John seemed to perk up; yet, sometimes he was more depressed after the call than he had been before. He was especially frustrated that his older son, Jamie, continued to teach in a rural Montana high school rather than going into business or studying to be an administrator. It seemed to Olivia that father and son had argued all of Jamie's life about their differences in values and politics— Jamie emphasizing independence and helping others and John insisting that a man also must be concerned about increasing his economic resources and his authority in the community. In spite of these differences, it was Jamie on whom they both counted to be there when his parents needed him.

Several months after John's hospitalization, Olivia saw their internist about the aches and weakness she was experiencing in her hands and back. She was given a prescription for a pain reliever and some exercises intended to strengthen both her back and her hands. Following this advice improved her condition, although she still had some difficulty buttoning her clothes and putting on her earrings. Since she didn't "dress up" much anymore, these were not major problems for her. She did enjoy reading and doing counted cross-stitch. The needlework gave her something to do while she watched TV with John, although she found that it gave her a headache to switch her eyes back and forth between the two.

One morning Olivia woke to find John missing from his place in their bed. After realizing he was not in the bathroom, she went to the kitchen to see if he had decided to fix coffee. Not seeing him there, she checked the other rooms and still could not locate him. When Olivia returned to the bedroom to get dressed so she could check outside, she saw John on the floor on the far side of the bed. Since she could get no response from him, she called 911 for an ambulance. John was declared dead on arrival at the hospital, attributed to a massive heart attack. She phoned Jamie from the hospital and asked him to come. He said he would call his brother and sister and make arrangements to get there as soon as possible.

Since they had never really felt part of their new community in North Carolina, Olivia contacted their former pastor in Pennsylvania and asked him to conduct a memorial service there for John. John's body was cremated and buried in a cemetery not far from the Wilsons' former home. During the funeral preparation and the service, Olivia was sustained by her long-time friends and her children. Not until the burial was over and her children returned to their own homes, did Olivia's deeper mourning begin. She was surprised to feel so angry with John for not protecting his own health and for leaving her feeling so helpless about their financial situation. The anger Olivia felt caused her to feel guilty and depressed.

Eventually, Olivia's anger, guilt, and depression became less frequent. She began to allow herself to enjoy her memories of the good times with John and their love for each other, although she still struggled with tears when these memories caught her in public settings. She often recalled the helpful words of Eda LeShan, "Our lives would be much less without our ghosts....To lose someone we love is agony; to have had that love is precious beyond words."

Olivia's grief for John was mixed with frightening concerns for her own future. John's death at age 68 had left Olivia at 66 feeling alone in their new home and in a community of which she did not feel a part. What was she to do? What alternatives did she have? Friends urged her to return to Philadelphia. Carol suggested that her mother move to a condominium development close to her family in Connecticut. Several months after John's death, Olivia decided to sell the home they had built and to buy a condominium in a complex in the Philadelphia area where two of her widowed friends lived. Her children agreed to take some of the furnishings she and John had moved to North Carolina, and within several months after John's death she returned to the familiar area.

Olivia did not resume her community roles and eventually stopped attending her former church. It seemed too far from her condo and she disliked the new minister's preaching style. She never became active in a new church, although she and another woman living in the condo complex occasionally went together to a nearby church for special services. Olivia gradually made some new friends, mostly women. One of the women in the condo complex whom she had known in earlier years soon moved to a nursing home, and other friends suffered from chronic problems. Some complained a good deal.

Olivia filled her days as well as she could by volunteering as a nursery helper at the hospital where John had once practiced, playing bridge with both old and new friends, and continuing with her reading and needlework. She also tried to resume the walking schedule she started initially to encourage John to exercise, but gave it up when she found the weather in Pennsylvania less conducive to regular walks than the weather in North Carolina. She also felt sad and lonely walking in the rain or snow by herself.

Two years after John's death, she was invited to travel with new friends on a European tour. Suddenly, Olivia had a sense of urgency about living life as actively as possible before it was too late. She decided to go. The projected expense prompted Olivia to get an updated assessment of her financial situation. While she knew that she had taken a loss in order to sell the North Carolina home quickly, only then did she realize that their brokerage account had declined rather than increased in value. In addition to living as they wished in retirement, Olivia and John had often talked about helping with their grandchildren's first home purchases, although they never made specific arrangements to do so.

On the recommendation of Carol's attorney husband, Olivia contacted a financial planner who helped set up an investment and annuity plan and a grandchildren's trust account. She did take the European trip, but found the prices much higher than she expected. After her "European fling," as Olivia called it, she found that shorter trips closer to home were better suited to her energy level as well as to her financial plan. For several years, she traveled each spring and fall with groups seeing the United States by bus and train, enjoying both the sites and meeting many interesting people.

As Oliva reached age 76, some 10 years after John's death, the arthritis in her back and hands was severe and affecting her knees as well. While she was still doing her own shopping and driving, her physician advised her not to drive at night. Her eyes no longer adapted quickly enough to changing amounts of light for her to adjust to either artificial light or bright sunlight driving conditions. Olivia stopped taking the group trips because she found it too difficult to do the climbing, long sitting, and light carrying which was involved. She was forced to give up her hospital volunteer work and her cross-stitch as well.

The best part of ending her travel period was that she could now have a cat to keep her company. John always preferred dogs and claimed he was allergic to cats, so she had not had one since childhood. Once she made her interest known to friends, she had several offers of kittens and adult cats who needed homes. Olivia eventually adopted a female, gray tiger-striped cat, about a year old, the pet of a woman who went to live with her son in another state. Olivia and her cat, Topaz, quickly became devoted friends who seemed to converse regularly about various subjects. Olivia's children claimed that she talked more about that cat than they did about their new grandchildren!

Increasingly, Olivia felt it required more effort than she could make to get ready to go someplace or prepare for someone to visit. Consequently, she spent many of her days alone, except for Topaz, either reading or watching television. Her telephone was a trusted tool that allowed her to visit with both her children's families and with her friends, most of whom were as "house bound" as she was.

When Carol made her annual visit, she realized that her mother had lost considerable weight during the year. Carol was also surprised by Olivia's limited activities and her declining confidence in what she could do for herself. Carol observed that Olivia had become set in her TV routine, to the extent that she ignored telephone calls and even visitors when watching certain shows.

There seemed to be little food in the house, and both the bathroom and the kitchen were badly in need of cleaning. She wondered how well her mother was handling her financial affairs, although she assumed that her broker, accountant, and attorney were checking on these matters. There were several different types of medication in the bathroom, apparently prescribed by various doctors for her eyes and for the pain of her arthritis. All of the prescriptions dated back to over a year ago when Carol knew her mother had her last physical examination. When she asked whether her mother was taking these medications regularly, she was not sure how to interpret Olivia's answer. In fact, she was not sure that her mother could recall when she took them.

Given this set of concerns, Carol called her brothers who agreed that it was time for them to assist their mother in considering either some type of care at home or some alternative living arrangements. Since Olivia had made her own decisions since their father's death, her children knew that they could only suggest and make information available to her. As far as they could tell, their mother was usually quite competent mentally, and they thought they could trust Olivia to make wise plans for the next stage of her life.

Key Issues for Olivia Wilson

It is too late for John Wilson to plan, although there were clearly some issues he might have addressed at various points during his years after 50. For example, John's lack of financial planning, his intense work and recreational styles, and his refusal to change his way of living and thinking were all issues which affected the quality, and possibly the number, of his final years. Without a doubt, John's attitudes and actions had a profound affect on Olivia, both while he lived and for the rest of her life as well.

The specific conditions now faced by Olivia Wilson:

- Physical limitations including severe arthritis, some loss of vision, and recent loss of weight;
- Uncertainty about the adequacy of her financial resources in relation to her possible needs for care in future years;
- Inability to drive safely at night or on bright days, limiting her independence;
- Evidence of declining attention to nutrition and use of prescribed medications;
- No local person responsible to either recognize or handle an emergency;
- Geographical distance from all three children making it difficult for them to work together to help with both planning and regular support;
- Family's lack of knowledge of alternative living options in the area where Olivia lives;
- Apparent continuing contacts by telephone and occasional visits with a number of friends;
- Continuing concerns for her on the part of her adult children; and
- Presence of Olivia's new pet.

Culminating Scenes

CHAPTER FOUR

"The riders in a race do not stop short before they reach the goal. There is a little finishing canter before coming to a standstill. There is time to hear the kind voice of friends and to say to oneself, 'The work is done.'"

—OLIVER WENDELL HOLMES, JR.

POIGNANT SCENES

Joe Swenson and Ruth and Peter Hereux are well into their 80s. All three have remained active and outgoing throughout their 70s, as more and more of us can expect to do. As octogenarians, they survived many of their friends, but have considerably more company in their age group than people in their 80s once did.

Each of these persons has experienced the loss of a spouse and has known a life rich with both joys and disappointments. Each one faces a very personal, often agonizing, decision about when to struggle against the physical and mental changes typical of those who have lived for eight decades and when to accept them as inevitable.

Freed from most of their earlier concerns about what

others expect of them, they find that memories and occasional regrets have replaced their dreams for the future. Life in the past frequently appears more satisfying, indeed more vivid, than life today or tomorrow. Telling their personal stories to family members and friends and finding ways to assure that they will continue to live on in some way have become compelling desires for them.

PROFILE #6

JOE SWENSON

> *"'You are old, Father William,' the young man said,*
> *'And your hair has become very white;*
> *And yet you incessantly stand on your head—*
> *Do you think, at your age it is right?'*
> *'In my youth,' Father William replied to his son,*
> *'I feared it might injure my brain;*
> *But now that I'm perfectly sure I have none,*
> *Why, I do it again and again.'"*

> —LEWIS CARROLL

Joe Swenson, age 83, has been a widower for several years and continues to live in Livonia, Michigan, close to Detroit. Joe and his wife, Lucy, had two children, John and Susie. Susie died in infancy, and her mother never quite recovered from the loss of her baby girl. John and his family live nearby, and Joe and Lucy regularly shared part of the holidays with them over the years.

Lucy had been ill often in the five years before her death and had few interests and little energy after she retired at age 65 from her bookkeeping job. Joe hadn't always been the "perfect husband" but he tried to interest her in the many activities he enjoyed and to plan outings and events she might like—perhaps to make up for the earlier times when he had failed her because of his attentions to other women. Lucy did seem to truly enjoy the fiftieth wedding celebration which John and his wife arranged shortly before her death after a stroke.

Joe has many friends and is physically active. He comes from a large family, and six brothers and sisters live in the Detroit area. Joe never seems to lack for companions to share his active life. The only job Joe ever held was on the assembly line at General Motors. He enthusiastically celebrated his retirement on his sixty-fifth birthday and plunged into doing what interested him most—swimming, hunting, and skiing with his buddies.

After Lucy's death, Joe became even more active in sports. He was free to go to hunting camp with his buddies in the fall and talked excitedly about the good times they had. Relatives suspected that killing deer interested Joe very little, but were glad that he enjoyed the outing and the camaraderie.

Throughout the year, Joe was an aggressive and winning contestant in senior swimming events. When you failed to reach Joe by telephone for a few days, you could assume that he was off participating in another swimming meet, and that he would report his winnings the next time you talked. Joe usually swam daily at the local YMCA pool to keep in shape for the contests and because he enjoyed it.

When the downhill skiing was good, Joe often missed swimming practice. Since he was past 80, he was permitted to ski free on weekdays, and he did so many times during the winter. His son and daughter-in-law worried that Joe would break his leg in a fall or catch pneumonia in the cold, but Joe persisted and looked forward to the coming winter season. Family members also realized that Joe's hearing was not good and that his short-term memory had failed. Since these changes occurred gradually, Joe himself was neither aware of nor bothered by them. Whenever someone suggested that he slow down, Joe retorted, "Age is nothing to a live man," a saying by Edward E. Purinton that he had once read in a sports magazine.

When Joe was 81, he experienced a difficult winter. First, a kitchen fire started when he left home for a weekend without turning off a gas burner. He had done that before when friends were around and admitted that he could not always remember whether or not he had done something. Later, a storm knocked out the power to his house for several days during unusually cold weather.

Joe thanked his son for the invitation to move in with them until the power was restored, but he refused to stay with them. Two weeks later, Joe was in the hospital with pneumonia, apparently because of living in the unheated house rather than being out on the ski slopes. His recovery was slow, and he watched TV for hours at a time, since he had always found reading hard work and not very enjoyable.

Joe didn't tell anyone, except one sister, how lonely and isolated he felt during the winter months when he could not get out to be with his friends. Their visits to him were infrequent. Because of concerns for what might happen to his father, John tried to get Joe to consider either moving in with one of his sisters or moving to a retirement home. By spring, Joe had returned to swimming and would not even discuss the possibility of moving from his home.

That summer, Gerald, one of Joe's swimming friends, died suddenly from a heart attack he suffered as he climbed from the pool after practice. Harry, another friend with whom Joe had often gone to hunting camp, became so confused and frail that his family arranged for him to move into a nursing home. Joe visited him there, but realized sadly that his friend of many years did not even recognize him. Early in the fall, Joe's older brother, Eric, had a stroke while driving and had to be hospitalized, then placed in a nursing home because he required assistance with eating and dressing. These losses were difficult for Joe, although he remained optimistic and planned his autumn hunting trip and put the senior swimming meet dates on his calendar.

In October, Joe received a call from Hiram, a younger man with whom Joe had once served as a volunteer fireman. Hiram reported that they were looking for someone who could tell them about the early years of the fire department before it had a full-time force, and hoped Joe would help with the project. At first Joe said that he was not the right person for the job; yet, as they talked, Joe realized that he remembered clearly some of the other men and the fires they had fought together 50 and 60 years ago— although he could not recall what he had done yesterday.

Hiram wanted to stop by the following week to talk with Joe and asked if he would mind if he brought a recorder to tape some of Joe's recollections. Joe agreed, but still worried that he would not be able to be helpful in this unfamiliar role. For several months, Joe, Hiram and other former volunteer firemen got together every few weeks to share their stories, often drinking beer and eating popcorn as they talked.

Occasionally, some of the wives and female friends accused the men of forming a club and reminded them that it was not fair to keep women out. Some of the men laughed, but others claimed this was serious business, not just partying. Whichever it was, Joe found that he anticipated each get-together and was sorry when Hiram said that he had enough material for the report he was writing. Some of the older men talked about continuing to meet, but nothing ever happened, probably because no one took responsibility for planning it.

After his difficult winter, Joe had gradually returned to swimming, hunting, and skiing, although his previously active friends seemed to be retiring rapidly from sports either because of death, illness, or moves to be nearer their children. Joe's Chevy was not new, but it had always been reliable, and he continued to drive everywhere he wanted to go. His health was reasonably good as long as he stayed active. When he did not vigorously exercise for several days, he found that his body argued with him when he tried to be active once again. It was increasingly difficult for Joe to keep active, however, since he had trouble finding someone else to exercise with and his own muscles protested after "taking time off."

Joe worked hard to stay in touch with his remaining relatives and friends, calling on their birthdays and going to visit those not too far away—a task he had taken over after his wife's death. He was more apt than they to remember such events; however, Joe had never been judgmental of others and did not let their occasional lack of thoughtfulness bother him. John and his family continued to stop by and invite him to share dinner when they could. These times were fewer than in earlier years, since John now worked two jobs; his wife was working full-time; and the children were busy with either high school or college.

Previously an early riser, Joe now slept late and dozed in his chair in front of the television late into the night. Since he used to swim in the mornings, he found it difficult to get in regular practice at the few periods when the pool was available later in the day. If John asked about his meals, Joe could seldom recall when or what he had last eaten.

Talking on the phone with Joe was frustrating, because he either didn't understand or could not accurately hear what others were saying. Joe's sister claimed he was "losing his marbles" rather than his hearing, because he often argued with her about things she had not said or talked about something she hadn't been discussing. Since she had always talked too much and was now 87, it was a bit difficult for others to figure out who had the greater problem.

During the fall of his eighty-second year, none of Joe's buddies went to hunting camp, so he did not go. That winter, only one of his senior friends continued to swim competitively, and icy roads kept them from two of the bigger meets. Worst of all, the corporation managing the mountain resort where Joe had previously skied declared bankruptcy and shut down all activities in mid-January before there had been any really good snow days. In spite of his own conviction that he was as physically fit as ever, Joe found himself sitting in the house watching TV and eating mostly "fast food." When he did see friends or family, Joe said that his active life was over and occasionally mentioned that he would probably die soon. Even though Joe seemed to want to talk about death, friends and family members generally changed the subject.

Either his younger sister or John's wife brought in food every few days—sometimes on the same evening. Joe would thank them, eat one helping, and promise to eat the rest later. But as far as they could figure, he seldom ate it later, because in future visits they would often find spoiled food on the counter or in the refrigerator. Planning meals ahead did not seem to work for Joe, since he failed to remember what food was available. He found it easier to drive for a pizza or burger when he felt hungry.

Concerned about Joe's weight gain and the changes in his exercise and eating habits, John insisted that his father see Dr. Adams, their family physician. John explained to the doctor before the exam how Joe had been living. Amazed to learn that he had gained 50 pounds since his last examination, Joe listened attentively when Dr. Adams recommended that he move into an assisted care home nearby, where he would be provided with three meals daily and would have others with whom to talk and share activities. The doctor said that Joe's heart was good, he seemed to have no severe digestive or urinary problems, and his active life and heredity had been good to him. Dr. Adams emphasized that Joe needed other interests beyond eating and watching TV at this stage of his life.

Joe agreed to go with John to visit the assisted care home the physician mentioned and learned that he could still keep his own car, could go out when he wished, and could bring personal furnishings for his room. Although he was polite during the visit, Joe angrily announced to John as soon as they returned to the car that he was not going into a nursing home and would die in his own home in control of his own life to the end. Nothing anyone said could convince Joe that the assisted care home offered a variety of activities for living and was not just a place for "crazy" or bedridden people to die.

Over the next few months, Joe became more withdrawn. When his sister or John visited, he talked mostly about his boyhood on a Michigan farm and his escapades in high school. He often commented that John's youngest son Mark, a "C" student, but a varsity football player, was just like his old grandad and would have a successful life just as Joe had. While Joe had always been fond of his two granddaughters, he now had trouble remembering their names and showed little interest in them. John was especially troubled by Joe's frequent references to the nearness of his death; yet he sometimes wondered if talking about death was his father's way of coming to terms with its inevitability.

Clearly, conditions had changed for Joe. His cheerful, active lifestyle had changed to a sad and sedentary one. There did not seem to be any medical reason why Joe could not live pleasurably and productively for more years if he changed his habits. Yet, before Joe's life improved, he himself would have to see and believe this.

How are those who love him going to help him understand this? How can they support Joe during this painful scene of his long and otherwise happy life? Is Joe saying to them that he is ready to die and that he plans to do it his way?

Key Issues for Joe Swenson

Joe Swenson, previously a physically active man, has become sedentary and backward-oriented in his eighty-third year. His family members see a number of issues that they believe should be addressed in order for Joe to live the next scene of his life as fully as possible. Joe, on the other hand, may see different issues as well as different resolutions. In general, key issues are:

- Loss of numerous friends because of death or severe incapacity;
- Continuing decline of short-term memory to the point of affecting healthy living;
- Poor hearing;
- Increasing withdrawal from others, and some complaints about his own loneliness and isolation;
- Rapid weight loss;
- Reduced opportunities to engage in activities he once enjoyed;
- Pleasure in sharing stories of his past;
- Personal history of being a positive and physically active man;
- Record of caring for both friends and family;
- Negative attitude toward assisted living options; and
- Frequent mention of his own death.

PROFILE #7

PETER AND RUTH HEREUX

"My glass shall not persuade me I am old,
So long as youth and thee are of one date;
But when in thee time's furrows I behold,
Then look I death my days should expiate."

—WILLIAM SHAKESPEARE

"Old age approaches, an awful specter of loneliness
to those who have never found joy in being alone."

—DOROTHY THOMPSON

We first meet Peter and Ruth Hereux late in their lives. Peter, age 86, was married for nearly 50 years to Susan prior to her death 10 years ago. Ruth, now 81, lost her first husband, Carl, suddenly when she was in her late 60s. Peter has three grown children, several grandchildren and great grandchildren, none living nearby. Ruth has four children, also with families of their own. One of Ruth's daughters lives nearby with her husband. In order to reassure their children and to keep matters straight between them, Peter and Ruth signed a prenuptial agreement intended to keep separate any assets each one brought to their marriage.

For several years, Peter and Ruth spent November through April in Sun City, Arizona, and the remainder of the year in Ruth's small home town in Ohio. Their life together has been quite happy, considering that they were lonely and felt isolated from social life after the deaths of their spouses. Both formerly enjoyed golf, but they played very little after they were married. Instead, they ate dinner out often and joined friends for cocktails whenever they could arrange it. Social life in Sun City was full, especially after Ruth was discovered by a group of Ohio State University alumni as the grandmother of the current quarterback. Not surprisingly, that set of relationships ended as suddenly as it had begun after their grandson graduated.

Peter had lost interest in playing cards, although Ruth was an avid player of both solitaire and bridge. He regularly read two newspapers and several business and news magazines in order to keep up on political and financial trends. Peter also liked to watch morning and evening TV news programs. Ruth was more interested in comedy on television. Peter also liked to watch basketball on TV, and they both enjoyed golf and football. Ruth had once been an active gardener and had numerous craft hobbies, although she did little of either after she and Peter were married. Visits from their children and grandchildren were welcomed, as long as they were brief. They recognized that neither took the place of the deceased parent for the other's children. Still, relations were cordial, and both sets of families seemed glad that Peter and Ruth were keeping each other active and alert.

At the time of their marriage, Ruth had sold her apartment in Sun City and moved into the home originally owned by Peter and Susan. When they decided to spend the spring and summer in Ohio, they jointly bought a condominium. Each contributed to a joint household account. Peter and Ruth kept their cars in their own names and replaced them as they wished.

After Peter's retirement from banking at age 65, he found great satisfaction in managing his own retirement investments, using his own somewhat erratic approach. On the conservative side, he kept a large percentage of his assets in a bank money market account. By contrast, he bought and sold both property and securities with frequency, using a number of different persons as his advisors or agents. Only Peter seemed to know what these assets were at any point in time, since he kept his records in a script which few were able to read. Ruth had taken a large loss on some risky stocks her first husband bought just before he died. Now one of her grandsons, an Ohio stockbroker, managed her assets.

During the last five years, Peter had suffered a series of health problems. Each round of problems seemed to begin with a medical mini-crisis of some type causing a few days of great concern for both Peter and Ruth and Peter's children. Then, he would be careful of his habits for awhile before slipping back into his established patterns of life—cocktails, smoking, irregular use of his prescriptions, primarily sedentary activities, and eating what sounded good to him. By the time he was 86, these mini-crises seemed to occur very close together.

First, he had urinary problems leading to prostate surgery but, fortunately, no cancer was found. Then, he experienced several respiratory infections from which he found it difficult to recover. Next, he had cataract surgery on the right eye and then on the left. Peter was disappointed when he found that his eyesight improved little, indeed it gradually seemed to worsen. He was supposed to use eye drops to prevent glaucoma, but the three-times-daily prescription was difficult to remember and to apply. He wore glasses to read, as he had done for years.

In recent months, Peter had lost considerable weight and found himself quite weak, to the extent that he feared falling down the stairs or tripping in the house. He resisted using a cane for some time, but finally agreed to do so and felt more secure. The diabetic condition which had first been diagnosed when he was 55 had always been kept under control by diet. Peter hadn't had a blood sugar test for some time; however, he and Ruth both knew that diabetes could affect his eyes as well as his general condition.

In spite of these problems, relatives joked that Peter's hearing was so good that you needed to be careful about what you said in a neighboring state for fear he would pick it up. Peter insisted that his mind was also in excellent shape, although his children agreed among themselves that his short-term memory had failed. He would tell each of them something several times and, to his children's considerable frustration, would come to different conclusions from one time to the next on a matter that they thought had been settled.

Ruth prided herself on being in excellent health and had little contact with physicians after she "conquered" menopause 28 years earlier. She wore glasses regularly and had the lenses upgraded every few years. If her eyes were weakening, she was not troubled by the change, since she no longer did the crafts she formerly enjoyed and never did much reading. Although she once enjoyed giving large dinner parties and cooking for family celebrations, Ruth seldom cooked a big meal anymore. She often picked up prepared food at the grocery or deli unless they ate out. Ruth admitted to her daughter that food just did not interest her much anymore, since she did not enjoy its taste as she once had.

Ruth, like Peter, had lost quite a bit of weight recently, but she said that she was glad to have an excuse for some new clothes. She often joked that her mind wasn't any worse than it had ever been and that her children and Peter had better not try to "put anything over on her." Ruth did most of the driving now because Peter's eyes failed to adjust from bright to dark conditions fast enough for him to see well either in the daytime or at night.

The summer that Peter was 85 and Ruth 80, Ruth was in a minor automobile accident that apparently resulted in a slight concussion, as well as a very sore back for several weeks. Neighbors and a niece and nephew who visited soon after her accident reported to Ruth's children that she sometimes seemed confused. The dizziness returned unexpectedly from time to time, so Ruth just took some of the pills her doctor prescribed after the accident. During Ruth's recovery period, it became obvious to those who saw them that Peter had become dependent on Ruth's management of their household as his own strength and eyesight had declined. Their independent lifestyle just did not go smoothly unless Ruth was fully well.

When Peter's two sons came to Ohio with their wives for a visit several weeks after Ruth's concussion, they were quite concerned about the changes in their father's capabilities and about the situation in general. They noticed that both Peter and Ruth wore the same clothes the entire weekend of the visit and that their always fastidiously groomed father had spots on his trousers and buttons missing from his shirt. There was little food in the refrigerator, and dirty laundry seemed to lie everywhere.

Garbage bags were piled in the garage and did not appear to have been taken to the dumpster in weeks. Peter's sons disposed of the garbage, made minor repairs, and suggested some changes intended to make the condominium safer and more comfortable. Unfortunately, the brothers' efforts to talk with their father and stepmother about the possibility of either getting regular household help or moving into a retirement community met with resistance. "We have a right to be where we're happy," "That's only for people who are 'over the hill,'" or the subject "can be discussed later" were the usual excuses.

In early Fall, Peter's daughter was surprised when she made her weekly call to learn that Peter was in the hospital recovering from surgery. After she contacted him there, he reported that he had had surgery on his leg intended to correct his unsteady walk and had not wanted to bother his children with the information ahead of time. He planned to return home as soon as possible to rest in bed most of the time while Ruth cared for him until he could be "up and around." Through a series of telephone conversations among Peter, Ruth, and Peter's three children, it was made clear to the children that they were not expected, or even invited, to come to Ohio. Peter's older son was especially insistent that they have a visiting nurse or home health aide. Since Peter's physician also advised such care for a few days, a home health aide came to assist. Several weeks later, Peter's son learned that Peter and Ruth had fired her before the first week ended because she seemed lazy and they felt her presence intruded on their privacy. Later, a neighbor agreed to come in and clean one day a week, but she took a full-time job after a month, so that arrangement ended. It seemed that all the children could do was to call more often and try to stay in touch to make sure that Peter and Ruth were still answering the telephone.

Over the next few months, three grandchildren went out at different times—each aware that these were final months or years for their grandfather. They tried to observe conditions, help as they could, and encourage their grandfather to consider either getting some help at home or moving to a retirement community. Karen, who had not seen her grandfather in two years, was shocked at Peter's loss of both weight and physical strength. Karen managed while she was in Ohio to round up some of the dirty clothing and do a washing under the pretense that her young daughter needed clean clothes.

After the Hereux's marriage, Peter managed both his own investments and their joint financial business. When his grandson, Drew, came to visit, he noted that Peter could no longer see to write his own checks and that Ruth was writing them and directing Peter where to put his signature. Sensing that these checks did not get listed in the check register regularly, the grandson asked about it only to be told that his grandad "has lots of money in the bank and it was, therefore, not a problem." Drew asked about Peter's investments and suggested that he himself found it helpful to have most of his investments in one family of funds and managed by a financial planner. He wasn't sure how his grandfather felt about that idea for himself, although he was informed that Ruth's grandson, a broker in another city, was handling some of Peter's investments.

When a third grandchild, Cary, visited and found little food in either the refrigerator or the cupboards, he asked how they handled their meals. He realized that his grandfather could no longer see well enough to prepare his own breakfast and snacks as he once had. Peter only ate what Ruth liked and had in the house, which seemed to be very little. Ruth said that her daughter or a neighbor often brought food, more than they could ever eat, so she threw out much of it. Ruth reminded them that the delicatessen had good prepared foods which she often bought for them.

When Cary discovered that the microwave, on which they presumably depended to heat such food, did not work at all, he purchased a new one and made sure that Ruth knew how to use it. Ruth was enthusiastic about Cary's suggestion that they have a fire in the fireplace and said she would open the damper. That lead to a new discovery—the fireplace flu was clogged and the batteries had been removed from the smoke detectors. Cary fixed these problems and pointed out that it would not be safe to remove the batteries again.

Even after Peter's leg improved to the point that he could use a walker, he generally declined invitations to the homes of relatives and friends and no longer went out to eat. Poor eyesight and general frailty seemed to be the reasons. The fact that he could no longer drive seemed to bother Peter more than any other single change. He expressed in several ways that he felt the loss of both social status and independence because he could not drive.

Ruth, always very socially active, lost contact with most

of her friends still living in the area and did not leave the condominium, except to go to the grocery store or to have her hair done. She said that Peter needed her, but she seemed to have no place to go. They both spoke of how much they cared for each other, yet showed increasing signs of being irritated with each other. They kept their church membership in Sun City, although it seemed unlikely they would return there, and they had not attended a church in Ohio. Both Peter and Ruth complained separately to different relatives that they felt very isolated from other people and often found the other quite difficult.

In the meantime, the frequent phone calls among Peter's children continued. There were a few contacts between one of Peter's sons and two of Ruth's children about the general state of things at the Hereux household. Ruth's children clearly did not want to irritate her by seeming to be interfering, although they also reported that they were in frequent telephone communication with both Ruth and Peter. Some of Ruth's children indicated concern about their independent living situation shortly after her fall during the summer; however, since her confusion seemed to have ended, they were less concerned about her staying in her own home, but shared the views of Peter's children that Ruth needed relief from the responsibilities of caring for both Peter and the household. Efforts to discuss getting help only irritated Ruth. In fact, she responded as if those who asked were questioning her abilities and rights, rather than being helpful.

Peter's children agreed that their father's health would be improved by an early move into some type of assisted living community, although they did not all share the same view of what type of community might be best. Peter himself seemed to be open to the possibility of such a move a few months into the future. There was no measurable progress toward arranging for management of Peter's finances now that he could not see to do so himself, although he said Ruth had found a young accountant to help in preparing their taxes.

For a few weeks after his older son offered to help oversee the bank accounts and suggested that Peter arrange for consolidation of his investments, there were signs of great anger and defensiveness. At one point, Peter made it clear that he trusted his wife more than he did his children and that they had better be careful how they treated her. The son was hurt by Peter's reaction and refrained from offering help for awhile. Even after relations seemed to improve, Peter stated from time to time that he was not going to let his children tell him what to do.

Ruth alternated between saying that she had friends in the retirement community and would enjoy being there, but at some later date, and admitting that she did not want to give up her home. She repeated both her agreement and her dissent frequently and, sometimes, angrily. This pattern of repetitious, but inconsistent behavior was typical of many of her of actions at this point. Previously, she and Peter had managed not to be depressed at the same time, but they both became discouraged when they learned that the surgery on Peter's leg had been unsuccessful, apparently because of his general physical condition. They each had to come to terms with the fact that Peter could never again do some things for himself because of his health.

Peter's options were either to complain and regret his loss of meaningful life as he had known it for 86 years or to learn how to live satisfactorily within his limitations of movement and vision during his final years. Sometimes he said that he could not go on much longer. Ruth had to deal with the fact that her future social life did not include an active, independent spouse and that either she or professional helpers would need to help care for his basic needs for the rest of his life. In her bitterness, Ruth even chided

Peter in front of family members about their lack of sexual relations, a subject she had cheerfully alluded to as exciting in their early years together.

While both Ruth and Peter had been treated for their medical emergencies, neither could recall having had a complete physical examination in a few years. Nothing their children said could get them to make and keep such appointments. Ruth also had her own continuing aging process to consider. Planning for their remaining years was sorely needed at this juncture, but both lacked the energy and focus needed to do this final planning alone. As Peter and Ruth fought to stay independent and in control of their lives, they probably did not think of the struggles in theological terms; however, they had come to the time in their lives when they each needed to experience the grace of receiving significant help from others.

Key Issues for Ruth and Peter Hereux

Identifying and dealing with the future needs of Peter and Ruth is complicated by the fact there are two groups of responsible family members and two sets of family relationships and practices. Key issues at this stage seem to be:

- Multiple physical problems for Peter, e.g., prostate condition, respiratory infections, diabetes, loss of vision, feebleness, and considerable weight loss;
- No known chronic physical problems for Ruth, except some weight loss and occasional dizziness;
- Need for physical examinations for both to verify and complete the information from the observations of family members;
- Poor household management, including providing for the basic needs of nutrition, cleanliness, and safety;

- Lack of knowledge on the part of family members about the adequacy of Peter and Ruth's financial resources and the quality of their financial management;
- Reduced social contacts within the community;
- Increasing short-term memory loss causing inconsistency and confusion for both Peter and Ruth;
- Reluctance to change their living arrangements coupled with differences between members of Ruth's family and Peter's about the urgency of doing so;
- Need for information about assisted living options in the area;
- No indication of advanced directives or plans for medical care in cases of terminal illness or death.

Planning the Next Scenes

CHAPTER FIVE

"I know now that one must plan one's old age as surely as one plans any other stage of life."

—ELIZABETH FORSYTHE

PLOTS WITH COMMITMENT,
CHALLENGE, AND CONTROL

Life's transitions to new scenes seldom catch us entirely by surprise. The stories in the previous chapters remind us that throughout our lives we face both expected and unanticipated transitions, most of them normal experiences for men and women in our society. Some of these transitions are caused by one major event, such as a diagnosis of cancer or retirement from a position. Other transitions are the result of multiple smaller changes which pile up until they become one big challenge. A few transitions are actually caused by nonevents—things that do not happen when we expect them to. For example, your hearing fails to improve after surgery to correct the problem, or the house you expect to sell quickly continues to stay on the market.

As teenagers and young adults, most of us developed the ability to picture ourselves in the next scene because we knew others who preceded us. In the teenage and early adult years, we enjoy imagining ourselves in the next scene because each one promises to be more exciting or rewarding than the last. We are eager to graduate from high school or college, become economically independent from our parents, get married, have children, live in our own homes, and, eventually, have the children leave home. As the years pass, our thoughts may turn to the possibilities of selling the family home, traveling, experiencing physical changes, and ultimately, to death. For most people, these scenes are mixed with sadness and joy. Some may offer rewards but, increasingly, the scenes can appear unpleasant, even frightening, to us.

While most adult transitions are age related, more importantly, these changes mark progress through the dramatic scenes which constitute each person's life. These individual transitions occur in relation to our external circumstances or special environments and also according to the internal conditions—personality and biological factors unique to each of us.

In spite of the normality of adult transitions, it seems to be human nature to put off conscious planning for the most important aspects of our lives as we age. Yet, many of us enjoy planning in certain ways. Some enthusiastically tackle planning a garden, redecorating the house, taking a trip, or giving a party. Others spend their working years helping others to plan and make key decisions about relationships, education, health, housing, religion, or finances. Unfortunately, we often fail our families and ourselves by neglecting to schedule the time, assemble the information, and use the decision-making strategies required to manage our own lives well. Still, don't we all want to "age well"?

Professionals who work with the elderly use the specific vocabularies of their fields to describe the conditions that typify those who age well. Different vocabularies aside, they all agree that aging persons require:

1. a sense of control over their own lives;
2. a sense of purpose and meaning for their lives; and
3. knowledge and skills for adapting to the inevitable challenges and losses of life.

While most teenagers and adults have needs related to control, commitment, and challenge, those of us in Act III have increasingly greater difficulties in all three areas as we age, perhaps because of the nature of the transitions we must make. What do control, commitment, and challenge mean to those of us in the Third Act?

COMMITMENT

Typically, newly retired women and men and often their spouses, give up volunteer roles at about the same time as they leave paid employment. By this point, those who are parents traditionally have launched their children into their own lives, even if some continue to live at home. These substantial changes in work, community, and parental roles result in a loss of commitment or sense of purpose for many of us. Suddenly, we may find ourselves without a focus for our lives, often combined with the feeling that no one needs or appreciates us. We are remarkably like we were as teenagers, asking, "Who am I, and what is the meaning of life?" Fortunately, we have gained experience and skills in addressing such questions, if we will only permit ourselves to do so. Nevertheless, after we work through satisfying answers to these questions at age 50 or 60, these answers may not suit us at 70 or 80. Consequently, we need to deal repeatedly with these purpose or commitment issues as part of our plot line in various scenes throughout Act III.

CHALLENGE

The years after 50 offer most men and women a better balance of work, play, and love than we have ever known. Nevertheless, amid the new joys and freedoms of mature life are difficult problems and losses. When we grew into adulthood, many of us were less aware than some of today's young people are of the pain and failure of relationships, careers, health, and finances that adulthood inevitably brings. Whatever our earlier optimism, aging adults can sometimes feel that life is just one loss or deficit after another—physical health, social contacts, role status, financial security, loved ones, mental stability, familiar surroundings, and finally, life itself. For almost all people, life after 50 becomes a challenging social, psychological, and biological process. Some never succeed in finding the positive challenges that could enervate or, at least, satisfy them at this point in life.

CONTROL

During a few difficult scenes of Act III, the pervading theme seems to be a steady loss of independence and power. As these changes occur, we risk losing the third essential ingredient to a healthy life, our sense of personal control. Yet, scenes dominated by loss are often followed by scenes of hope and new pleasures. Clearly, each aging person must deal continuously with commitment issues and must manage the successive challenges of life in order to maintain a sense of being in control. We cannot fully control—or even precisely predict—what challenges we will face; however, each of us can develop strategies and take steps toward controlling how we will respond to our challenges.

As we note in the stories told in earlier chapters, managing ourselves as aging persons can be complicated by the fact that our children, spouses, and close friends are also struggling with their own transitions. Adult children have complex responses to their parents' aging. It can be difficult for concerned daughters and sons to tell whether a problem reported by aging parents is primarily one of perspective and emotion or whether it is one that should be handled largely as a technical and procedural issue. It is helpful to determine before responding whether a given concern on the part of either parent or adult child is primarily one of relationship, such as facing changing family roles, or is a practical problem, like assuring adequate financial resources.

Most of us wish to spare our children from as many of these concerns about our aging as possible. Nor do we want our children or anyone else to manage our lives. Surely, these are compelling reasons for developing our own scripts for the mature years.

With this background, let us return to our characters as they plan the scripts for the next scenes in their diverse lives. As you read the continuing stories, ask yourself:

1. Which people are successful in maintaining control over their lives by managing the commitment and challenge tasks?
2. How do they make their decisions?
3. Which persons develop scripts for the next scenes that leave them with appropriate options for the rest of the act?
4. By contrast, why and how do some people seem to restrict their future roles unnecessarily?

SARAH AND JAMES ENDICOTT

You will recall that the Endicotts are considering whether or not James should take the early retirement package offered by his company. Remember also that this offer to James has come at a time when Sarah is apparently feeling fulfilled by her job, home, family, and community roles.

As James shares information about his retirement package with Sarah at their special dinner, they begin to discuss what this could mean for each of them. One or the other mentions the reduced income, the situations of their parents and their children, Sarah's paid and volunteer jobs, and concerns for their future health. As they talk over dinner, each becomes troubled by the other's apparently opposite reactions to the situation.

Sarah seems most threatened by James's ideas for selling their house and moving to a place where their expenses could be reduced. She feels as if some evil bird is about to take her from all she cared about only to drop her into some unfriendly, unknown world, where she would be forced to build a brand new nest. She points out that they had seldom taken long vacations, let alone considered living permanently in a different community. Furthermore, she does not understand why James would take the early retirement offer if he doesn't have to do so.

James, on the other hand, is stimulated by the prospect of such a change but is worried about the financial implications of early retirement. He feels that being free from the obligations of his job would be its own reward and that selling their house and making a move would become his new focus in life. After that is over, he will decide what to do with himself next. James is frustrated that Sarah seems unwilling to consider the unexpected opportunities early retirement provides. Why are they having such different reactions to their circumstances?

The next morning at breakfast, James comments that he hopes they can talk further that evening about the retirement offer, since he needs to give the company his answer soon. Both he and Sarah think a good deal about it during the day. When they begin to talk again, they agree that they are evaluating where they are; however, they also conclude that they are not sure how to progress toward the steps necessary to making the critical decisions required and to acting on those decisions. Since they found a professional counselor helpful when their marriage was threatened by James's affair, they decide to see a retirement planning counselor to help them get started.

Their counselor meets with them three times—first together, then separately, and lastly together. By the time they complete the sessions, they conclude that James should accept the early retirement offer, but that they will not sell the house right now. The sessions with the counselor also enable them to develop a list of the many issues and tasks they face and to agree on a process for dealing with each of them. Neither James nor Sarah is prepared to make decisions about the long term.

James tells his employer that he accepts the early retirement package, and his retirement date is scheduled for two months later. In the meantime, both Sarah and James consider in their own ways what adjustments they can make to the reduced family income and start thinking about handling the increased time available for James. While they occasionally talk briefly about their hopes and concerns for the future, this is a period of individual consideration rather than mutual decision making.

Sarah uses some of this time to talk with close friends and with their pastor about her feelings and to solicit suggestions. It is especially helpful to Sarah to talk with a friend whose husband retired two years earlier about the way in which their lives changed. Sarah also feels better after she shares some of her fears about James's retirement and the need to decide how to handle this matter with their two older children, Joan and Donald.

By nature a more private person, James finds the seminar and materials provided by the corporate consultant hired to assist those taking early retirement quite helpful in suggesting alternatives and additional resources. He locates some of the materials about financial planning, retirement housing, and health care in the local library and uses them to complement his own ideas about options for the future. He also directs their accountant to project three different income and expense scenarios for their consideration, based on high, low, and mid-range assumptions about future investment earnings and living expenses.

The Endicotts realize that it is fortunate they are not forced by either financial or medical emergencies to sell their house and move quickly when James enters retirement. As suggested by their retirement counselor, they take a brief vacation to visit friends in Florida after James ends his work with Ralston Purina. On returning home, they spend a scheduled period each week discussing what each has been thinking and feeling, a strategy they learned working with the retirement counselor. Over the span of several months, Sarah and James gradually develop the script for their next scene, hoping to leave the rest of Act III as open-ended as possible.

Taking on new roles and ending or revising existing ones renews and adds pleasure to their lives, although such transitions typically require that each person be unusually sensitive to their partner's feelings. Both James and Sarah try to address their own feelings and needs as well as adjust to each other's concerns. In doing so, they discover they're retaining some aspects of their previous lives, reducing others, and beginning to take on new activities and emphases.

The major continuation for both James and Sarah is remaining in their established home and community. They made that agreement with the understanding that they will reconsider the situation each spring in light of both housing market conditions and their personal situations. The implications of this decision are that when the selling price of houses in the area increases substantially or when they find they cannot manage comfortably in their home because of either financial or health reversals, they will sell and move. They agree to explore other locations in conversations with friends, through reading, and by visiting. In order to maintain their good health, they start a regular exercise walking program together, committing themselves to walking for at least one half hour three days each week, no matter how busy they are or how bad the weather.

Sarah decides not to continue her church leadership role for another year. Instead, she plans to pursue her developing questions about faith by joining a weekly study group at church. She likes to quote Janet Bonellie saying, "I've reached the age when I can't use my youth as an excuse for my ignorance any more." Although James never joins the group, he and Sarah discuss some of the ideas at home. He is particularly interested in some of the theological questions about life's meaning and individual responsibility that develop from the study.

Sarah also talks with the owners of the real estate firm where she works, requesting more flexibility so she can enjoy occasional travel with James and visits with her much anticipated grandchild. The partners are eager to retain her experience and competence, so they agree to let her work four days a week and take a month's vacation during the autumn season when business is slow. Sarah decides that it is wise for her to continue to study for her real estate broker's examination.

Joan's daughter, Elizabeth, is born during this transition

year for the Endicotts. Grandmother Sarah is planning stories, making frilly clothes, and talking of trips to the zoo before her new granddaughter even leaves the hospital! Sarah is delighted to keep Elizabeth for occasional weekends and is glad that Joan and her husband live only an hour's trip away. James at first has only a passing interest in his new status as a grandfather; however, by the time his granddaughter is six months old, he is convinced that she is the smartest baby he has ever seen. To his wife's surprise, he actually goes to stay with baby Elizabeth overnight when her parents want to attend a friend's wedding and Sarah has to be at work.

James begins to golf more regularly with some other recently retired partners. He enjoys this group of men, who are less competitive about their game and more congenial than his previous corporate golfing buddies. His golf scores actually improve as he relaxes, and he occasionally wins against one of his former opponents.

A few months after James retires, a friend who owns a small hardware store has to undergo major surgery. He asks James to "mind the store" for him, and James finds that he thoroughly enjoys dealing with both the business and the customers. During the months of the owner's recuperation from surgery, James helps regularly, improving the computerized inventory system as he works with it. James starts to consider having his own business, perhaps purchasing a franchise operation of some type.

By this time, Sarah and James agree to reduce their expenses as much as possible in the areas of clothing, household and yard maintenance, and gifts, in order to travel some and remain in their large house. While these reductions do not save significant amounts of money, they accommodate for inflation and provide some sense of financial control during an uncertain period in their lives.

Then, James's mother dies suddenly within a year after

her son's retirement. For a few months, James spends many hours each week on the execution of her estate. Sarah's parents continue to live in Arizona, but their less active lifestyle and growing complaints about their health and frequent requests for her to visit cause her to feel guilty and concerned. The Endicott's son, Donald, and his wife seem to be managing their marriage and jobs well. Their younger son, Paul, graduates from college and, to his parents' considerable relief, finds a job that allows him to support himself, although not at all in the fashion he had hoped. Sarah realizes that their responsibilities for family members could increase at any time in the near future. In the meantime, the new scene they have written for themselves is playing quite well.

JERRY AND MARIA RODRIGUEZ

Jerry and Maria Rodriguez weathered Jerry's recovery from open heart surgery and took steps toward turning their plumbing business over to their two older children. Maria suffered also during Jerry's illness and recuperation. In fact, she was starting to feel as if it was time for her interests and feelings to be primary for awhile. They decided that it was time to talk about completing the business transfer to their children and where they would live in the next period of their lives.

Before they had a chance to talk about their own plans, Maria's mother died in her nursing home in San Juan. During the family reunion after her mother's death, Maria reestablished close relations with a cousin living in Miami. Upon returning home, she announced to Jerry that it was time for them to move to Florida and begin the relaxed life for which they had worked so many years. She talked excitedly about buying a new house, inviting their children, grandchildren, and friends to visit, and just enjoying life.

Jerry attempted to slow her down a bit by pointing out that he still had full legal and financial responsibility for their business and that they had no idea where they might live in Florida or what type of house they could afford. It seemed that Maria expected this reaction from her husband and was prepared. She already has accepted an invitation to spend several weeks in Miami with her cousin, now that Jerry is well. She pointed out that she needed the rest and could also look for a house. In the meantime, he should make arrangements for the complete transfer of the plumbing business to Anna and Ortiz.

Both their daughter, Anna, and their priest commented that Jerry and Maria were moving very suddenly and that there were, perhaps, other possibilities, such as vacationing together in Florida to try out the different lifestyle. Nevertheless, within three months from their first conversation about making a change to Florida, Jerry and Maria became both inactive partners in their business and new owners of a house and pool in Miami. Anna and her husband contracted to buy her parents' house in Queens. Maria happily gave them her dark, heavy furniture and the formal drapes and made plans to furnish her new home with wicker and light fabrics. Over Jerry's protests, she even sold to a neighbor the big oak desk which Jerry bought when he set up the business in their home, claiming that it would be expensive to move and would not suit their casual Florida home.

After their move to Miami, Jerry tried to continue writing his stories. Ortiz suggested two magazines to which he might send them for possible publication. The stories he submitted were rejected by both publishers and Jerry did not "have the stomach" to risk further rejection. Without his grandchildren nearby to encourage him by their admiration or an interested publisher, Jerry soon lost interest in writing his stories.

He was relieved to get the monthly reports from Anna and Ortiz showing that the business was prospering. In some ways, though, it depressed him to know that they were doing so well without him. Financially, he and Maria were comfortable, but Jerry himself lacked energy and had difficulty either concentrating in the daytime or sleeping at night. He became less careful about his low-fat diet and neglected to develop a regular exercise plan to fit their situation in Florida, claiming that living in such a climate offered many chances for walking and swimming. Privately, however, Jerry was experiencing symptoms that caused him to fear new heart problems.

Maria delighted in buying her new furniture, ordering designer shades for the windows, and sitting by her pool drinking rum-laced fruit concoctions. She issued numerous invitations to their friends from Queens and to their children and grandchildren, but almost no one was able to visit them. When she tried to get acquainted with her Miami neighbors, she quickly learned that most were either black or of Cuban background, not Puerto Rican, and that they had little enthusiasm for becoming her close friends.

Eventually, Maria began to fall asleep early at night after sunning and drinking throughout the afternoon. When she did stay awake, she was likely to lash out at Jerry for not doing anything to make their lives more exciting and happy. Within several months, Maria gained 25 pounds as a result of these habits, adding shame about her appearance to her troubles. This scene was not playing well for either Jerry or Maria. They were on the way to a very unhappy, and possibly even abbreviated Third Act for one or both of them unless someone or something convinced them to end this scene and develop a new one. Why have they failed, and what can they do now?

SYBIL AND LARRY STINE

You recall that the Stines retired to an anticipated life of tennis and parties in Coral Gables a few years before Sybil suffered a crippling stroke. Their daily activities changed considerably, as had the ways in which they viewed each other and themselves. Since Sybil's hospitalization, they had been dealing with new challenges as they arose, but they had not discussed either their personal feelings or the future. After Jake's irritating challenge to his father about dealing realistically with approaching the mid-seventies, they finally began to talk.

While Larry and Sybil previously had many acquaintances, neither now had close friends other than each other. Both were initially very cautious in expressing the disappointment and anger they each felt about the situation in which they found themselves. It was relatively easy to list the external factors of their lives, such as their move to Coral Gables from Cleveland Heights, Sybil's stroke, and their sons' distant and busy lives; however, neither found it comfortable to tell the other of the personal fears and frustrations they had.

About this time, their son Jake sent a book which advised the use of a deliberate decision-making process to deal with the essential changes of life. The author also recommended that when two persons were involved in these changes a specific communications process be used to identify the issues which needed to be addressed. Neither Larry nor Sybil felt they required anything complicated, but they did decide to schedule times for each to tell the other of his or her concerns without interruption from the other. They tried to follow these communications of concern with brief periods of questioning and feedback and to avoid rebuttals.

Over the next few weeks they talked more openly with

one another than they had in years. By doing so, each felt more loved and at ease than they had before. Larry used his "talking times" to describe the challenges he felt and his sense of inadequacy in dealing with them. He gave Sybil his estimate of their financial situation, described what he knew about his prostate condition, and admitted how inept he felt in assuming the household tasks that his wife appeared to handle with ease. Larry also confessed that he lost much of his interest in strenuous tennis games and no longer enjoyed the occasional cocktail and dinner parties they now attended.

Sybil tried hard not to be too negative; however, it was difficult for her to describe without tears her deep sense of loss as a result of her stroke. She admitted that she had actually been lonely ever since their move. Sybil missed her former house and the established routines and contacts of their earlier life. In addition, she now felt deeply angry about the limited mobility of her body and the changes in her appearance. Her bitterness about their son Barry's divorce and his wife's not bringing the children to see her was aggravated by her regret that both sons continued to live such a long distance from them.

As Sybil and Larry described their sense of the situation, it became clear that both were ready to make some major changes. Admitting that their first decisions after retirement had not produced the results they had hoped for was difficult. Yet, they both decided that they must live for the present. As Knut Hamsun has said, "In old age…we are like a batch of letters that someone has sent. We are no longer in the past, we have arrived." They agreed that the next step was to develop some alternatives about where and how they would live in the next scene. Larry had used in business a technique he called "brainstorming" and suggested that they use a similar process. They first listed every place that appealed to either of them without comment. Then, they each spoke of every activity that interested them and listed those. Sybil's desire to live on a houseboat and Larry's dream to design and sell kites had them both laughing.

With Sybil's advice, Larry refined their list and eliminated the activities and locations which were not realistic in light of their deeper interests, their financial resources, or their health. They agreed that this time their choices of location and activities should meet their mutual needs to develop new commitments or purposes in their lives as well as to accommodate realistically their medical and financial conditions. They spent several evenings discussing these remaining alternatives.

Moving back to the Cleveland area initially seemed appealing to both of them, but they decided that many older friends were now moving away and that they really preferred a milder climate where they could garden during most of the year. Staying in Coral Gables was too expensive for them over the long term. Since they had not established deep roots there, now seemed the time to move. After several discussions, the alternative that continued to excite both Larry and Sybil was a smaller, less socially prestigious community in northern Florida where expenses would be lower and seasonal gardening could be done.

While they had visited friends in two such communities, they did not have all of the information they wanted before making a decision. Larry emphasized the cost of living and being close to a good hospital, while Sybil wanted to be certain that there were musical events available in the area. Both agreed that they needed a house on one level with favorable conditions for gardening. On this basis, Larry contacted realtors in both communities and described their needs. He also volunteered to contact their physicians to ask about medical resources in both areas. Sybil called the Chamber of Commerce in both towns to request packages of information. In addition, she began to list the household arrangements she either preferred or required because of her wheelchair confinement.

Within a few months, the Stines decided where to move and discussed their plan with both Jake and Barry by telephone. Their sons seemed relieved by the decision, and Jake offered to take some vacation time to help them move when they were ready. By this time, Sybil had contacted their long-time friends in the town where they were moving and received a warm welcome. Luckily, their condominium sold quickly. As they start off to their next life scene in northern Florida, both Sybil and Larry are nervous about making another change, but glad to be in control of their lives once again and starting new adventures.

BESSIE SMITH

When we left Bessie Smith, she had enthusiastically decided to invite all four of her children and other family members to spend the Fourth of July weekend in Pontiac. She wanted to discuss with them what she should do with herself following her hip surgery and other medical problems and the loss of her church role. She especially wanted to share a holiday celebration in her home with those she loved most.

In spite of their own financial and job concerns, Jennie, Joe, and Lavonna did come home to join Kevin and Bessie, bringing several children and grandchildren with them. Her numerous descendents seemed to be bursting out of Bessie's modest house, but she was overjoyed to have them all around her once again.

Late one evening, Bessie and her four children sat down around her kitchen table to listen to some of Bessie's ideas about what she should do next. By this time, she had said enough to each of them that they realized she felt she needed a new interest in life and that she was thinking about selling the house. Joe and Lavonna had taken Bessie to visit three different group homes for older women, one in Pontiac and two in nearby towns. Kevin had also confided to his older sister that he was HIV positive and that he planned to move in with his companion when his mother sold the house. Bessie had talked with an officer at her bank about her savings account and her pension from State Farm, so she would know how much she could spend each month. He advised her to plan for about a five percent increase in expenses annually, just to be safe.

With this background, Bessie's children were able to put concerns for their mother ahead of their own regrets about giving up the childhood home and urged her to move to a group home. It was painful for Bessie to think of Kevin's move away from her just when she thought he might need her most; however, he helped her to understand that he wanted to make the move and that she needed to do what was best for her now. Her children agreed, some rather reluctantly, that she had taken on their concerns long enough and that it was about time to begin to care for Bessie. They believed that her financial resources were enough to provide for her, but Jennie and Kevin especially understood that Bessie was going to need cheering up sometimes. Their mother always seemed to have enough faith and joy for all of them in earlier years.

It was very hard for Bessie to say "good-bye" to each of her children and their families. She had a sense that they might never all be together again until her funeral. Before she fell asleep that night, she read her Bible, searching for passages that would console and uplift her.

Still, she knew she had work to do to complete her plans and getting started with her next life scene. Now that she had decided to sell her home, she must make her final decision about where to live. Actually, she had never been very open to the idea of leaving Pontiac, so the private home in Pontiac was likely to be her choice. It was owned and managed by a couple she had known for many years through her church, so she felt comfortable with her choice for that reason as well.

Since Bessie's decisionmaking usually involved prayer and talking matters over with the pastor, she called Pastor Brown and scheduled a time to see him. He listened to her ideas, suggested that they pray together, and asked her what she thought she would do. By the time she left the church office, Bessie decided to move into the Pontiac home and to ask Kevin to work with her on a plan for selling the house and dividing up the family possessions.

Sorting her collections from family living over many years provoked numerous memories: sad ones about the loss of her husband and problems with the children, and humorous ones, also involving her husband and children. She discarded numerous items and papers, wondering why she had saved so many of the children's school papers and reports from church. Others she put into boxes for each of the children to take. She planned to move her bed, chest, special chair, and two lamps to her room in the group home. The children did not seem to want the rest of her furniture, so Kevin helped her organize a garage sale. They gave the remainder to Goodwill.

Although it was difficult to give up cherished things, Bessie felt remarkably less burdened. Even more important, bringing back the memories made her feel very satisfied with herself. She was proud of the work she had done as a wife, mother, employee, and church leader!

You will not be surprised to know that shortly after her move to the new home, Bessie started a prayer group with some of the women there and invited others from her church to join them. Guiding this new group gave Bessie opportunities to deal with her own spiritual questions and satisfied her social needs as well. Most days she truly liked sharing her meals with the other women in the home. And, she was relieved when she had a "setback" with her hip to know that she could expect help from the staff in doing her laundry and getting dressed.

While moving into her new group home did not keep Bessie from being concerned about her adult children, especially Kevin, she was glad she had made the decision to move and to simplify her life. She occasionally wished that she could still be in her own home and active in her previous church roles, but Bessie liked most of her new friends and was glad to be surrounded with caring people.

OLIVIA WILSON

Following her husband's death 10 years earlier, Olivia Wilson left their retirement home in North Carolina in order to return to the Philadelphia area. She made new friends, traveled, and did some volunteer work until arthritis and poor eyesight finally kept her confined to her condo and the companionship of her beloved cat.

On her annual visit, Olivia's daughter, Carol, found her mother very limited in her activities and concluded that Olivia, at age 77, should no longer live alone, especially since none of her relatives were nearby. Carol told Olivia that she should consider moving to a place where there would be other people like her who wanted the benefits of nursing care and help with daily tasks. Both Carol and Olivia agreed that staying in the condo and getting some-one to come in daily was a possibility, but would not pro-vide the social contacts that Olivia really desired.

Before Carol left town, she contacted the local Area Agency for the Aging and made arrangements for someone to visit Olivia weekly and notify Carol if specific assistance seemed to be required. She also phoned Jamie, her older brother, who volunteered to research retirement homes in the Philadelphia area, since they agreed their mother was not likely to want to leave the area again.

Jamie located several types of facilities. Some offered "Independent Living," much like Olivia now had, but with addtional housekeeping assistance. Others, referred to as "Assisted Living," provided private or shared rooms with meals, protective oversight, varying social activities, and personal care services, other than nursing services. Some were board and care homes called Congregate Care, which provided rooms, meals, and assistance with daily tasks as long as residents met specific health guidelines, often requiring that they be able to get around on their own and not be incontinent. Neither Jamie nor Carol thought Olivia should be in a nursing home, since her arthritis and vision problems did not normally prevent her from managing routine tasks. Her needs for daily contacts with other people and for nearby assistance in an emergency seemed to be the most critical. Carol indicated concerns about improving her mother's diet and use of medications.

Jamie's research lead him to consider the advantages of Continuing Care Retirement Communities (CCRC), several of which were in the Philadelphia area; some were called Life Care Communities. All provided services ranging from skilled nursing to housekeeping as specified by a contract, usually for the balance of the resident's life. Most offered apartment living, and a few also offered separate houses or condominiums. Both were designed for elderly persons and offered emergency buttons and special safety features in the kitchens and bathrooms. Residents were expected to have at least one common meal daily and had access to nursing care at no additional cost in cases of acute or chronic illness.

Jamie decided this type of place exactly suited his mother's condition and sent for information from the four that sounded most appropriate. He summarized the information he had assembled for his mother, brother, and sister, and Olivia agreed that these places sounded pleasant. Without further discussion with Olivia, Carol and her husband and brothers agreed that the Pine Knoll CCRC sounded best.

Carol's husband, a corporate attorney, was especially vocal about the need to make a firm decision now while they all were involved with the matter. The result was that they strongly urged Olivia not to rent an apartment in the Community, but to make the investment payment which would assure a fixed price and provide nursing care when it was needed at no additional housing cost. In the meantime, Carol's husband developed a financial plan which depended on Olivia's selling one-third of her assets to make the payment and buying an annuity with the remainder of the funds. The annuity payments would cover the monthly fee payments and Olivia's discretionary expenses. It would also name the three children as beneficiaries so that the money would go to them after their mother's death.

The whole plan seemed very structured and rapidly decided on to Olivia; however, she knew little about either financial management or retirement living options and appeared relieved to have someone else make these bewildering decisions. Jamie took his mother to visit Pine Knoll, located in a rural area about 10 miles outside of the suburb where she now lived. Although Olivia reported that she found Pine Knoll pleasant, she said she did not know what it would be like to live there. The most important matter to Olivia right now was that she could take her cat, Topaz. Olivia's condo sold within a few months, and she gave away or sold still more of her furnishings and mementos, as well as her car. At Pine Knoll, she would eat dinner in the dining hall and prepare her own breakfast and lunch in the kitchenette of her one-bedroom apartment. Carol talked enthusiastically to Olivia of the day trips, discussion groups, and the swimming therapy class, which her doctor said might help her arthritis. Her first day there was rather bewildering, but Olivia hoped that the routines would become more comfortable and that she would be able to learn her way around in spite of her limited vision.

Within days, Olivia called Jamie to say that she hated Pine Knoll and wished that her children had not made her move. All three children tried to stay in close touch with their mother, but did not know what to suggest or do to assist her. Olivia seemed to feel that she was not fully accepted by some of the other residents. This was particularly true of those who shared a background in the rather prestigious Episcopalian church nearby that sponsored the original development of Pine Knoll. Olivia herself had grown away from the unquestioning religious faith of her earlier years and had never been an Episcopalian.

For two unhappy years, Olivia struggled to make herself get up, get dressed, and limp to the dining room each evening. She tried the swimming class, but the swimming instructor seemed to become impatient with her; then, she caught a cold after the second class and never returned. Her physician said that her vision had stabilized and her arthritis should not prevent her from taking short trips or sitting for an hour or so in a discussion group, but Olivia never joined in either activity. She did sign up for a discussion group on folk art but, after she realized that the leader was planning to center all of the discussion around slides he was presenting, she dropped out. She could see little of what he was talking about.

Eventually, the Pine Knoll social worker called Jamie to report of staff concerns about Olivia. In summarizing the situation, she said that Olivia seemed depressed and withdrawn to the extent that she was not functioning well either by herself or with others in the dining room. Olivia was apparently sleeping most of the day and staying awake during the night. It was difficult for her to get to dinner on this schedule, and Olivia's all-night television was disturbing her neighbors. Both Jamie and Carol realized that Olivia was having trouble managing her checkbook and has over-drawn her account several times. All three of the children knew that their mother continued to be angry with them for "putting" her into Pine Knoll and leaving her no options because of the irreversible financial commitment. Olivia herself reported that even the cat was miserable, as evidenced by his recent refusal to use the litter box. There was undeniably a problem!

Carol's husband was tired of hearing about his mother-in-law's problems. This made it difficult for Carol to spend much time or money on Olivia's needs. Ken had not been close to his mother since he reached adulthood. Once again, it was Jamie who came out over the summer and spent 10 days visiting his mother and working with the professional staff to figure out what could help Olivia. He and the social worker concluded that what she needed was a new interest or purpose in life to get her excited about living again.

Jamie observed that Olivia stayed well informed by listening to radio, some TV, and a regular supply of music and books on tape provided by her family. Even prior to her move to Pine Knoll, she had missed having someone with whom to share the information and ideas she had. Maybe that would offer a clue for improving Olivia's view on life.

An answer seemed to be provided for two lonely people when a woman whose husband had recently died moved into the apartment next to Olivia's. The social worker introduced the two of them, and they seemed to enjoy each other. Later, the social worker asked Olivia to help her support this new resident in making the difficult dual adjustment to being both a new widow and a new resident of Pine Knoll. Olivia agreed to try and reported enthusiastically to

Carol about her new friend when she telephoned. There seemed to be promise of a new, happier scene for Olivia.

JOE SWENSON

By age 83, Joe Swenson has become sedentary and withdrawn compared with his previously active life in outdoor sports and social groups. While Joe's son, John, lives nearby and is attentive to his father, many of Joe's friends have either died or are ill. Joe is very lonesome, and his limited hearing and frequent memory loss add to his difficulties.

Joe's persistent mention of death as well as his obvious weight gain prompted John to talk with his father's physician once again. The physician recommended even more strongly than before that Joe move to a board and care home, where assisted living would support him. The physician pointed out that Joe did not now need 24-hour nursing care and that in-home services on a frequent basis would be quite expensive and sometimes were undependable. Joe's financial resources are too limited for him to consider a CCRC, although he has enough money to support himself at home. If and when Joe needs nursing care, his family expects to rely on Medicaid after Joe's funds are depleted.

Since Joe disliked the place they had visited earlier, John offered to locate and report to Joe about other possibilities. He learned in talking with a co-worker that his own company offered help to its employees who had care responsibilities for their parents and would even permit him to use a few daytime hours on company time to contact Assisted Living homes in the area. Using information from a brochure provided by the human resources department, John contacted several of the homes by telephone that were located either in or near Livonia. John also discovered that the local housing and community development office sometimes provided assistance in finding "assisted care," and other similar facilities.

After John found three places that sounded like reasonable choices, he told his father what he had learned and asked him to visit the three homes with him. Joe agreed to make the visits and liked two of the three places very much. On their visit to one home, Joe met a man with whom he had gone to hunting camp occasionally and another against whom he had competed in swimming. Both men described the meals as "great" and seemed to be happy to have someone else worry about the household tasks. Joe knew several women in two of the homes they visited who had moved in after they were widowed. Some of these people still drove their own cars, and most talked as if they had busy lives and often saw people who lived outside the home.

Joe decided that he was willing to live in such a place when the time came that he could no longer stay in his own home. There was a room scheduled to be available later in the month at Woodsview, but not in the other home that Joe had liked. John commented that Woodsview was just a block from the swimming pool where his father had formerly practiced regularly. Together the men completed initial application papers for both homes. While John believed that great progress had been made, it became clear as they completed the papers that Joe was resisting the move. They eventually agreed to file the applications in order to get on the waiting list for a later time rather than for the room currently available.

Less than a week later, John answered the telephone and heard his father's nearest neighbor report that Joe had just fallen on the ice as he went out to get his mail. The neighbor had called an ambulance and her husband had gone to cover Joe with blankets and to be with him until the ambulance arrived. John met his father in the hospital emergency room, both of them frightened and unsure of what next steps they would have to take. Although Joe did not seem to be badly injured, because of his age and possible shock, the emergency room doctor admitted him for at least overnight.

By the next day, it was clear that Joe had, amazingly, not broken any bones. The doctor commented that Joe's active life had probably made him much less susceptible to fractures than many people of his age. Nevertheless, Joe was very uncomfortable because of muscle strains and bruises. Moving around hurt, and Joe required John's help to dress for his return home.

As they drove to Joe's house, John offered to arrange for daily Meals-on-Wheels and said he would stop in each morning and evening to help Joe dress and do household tasks. Joe was relieved to see John the next morning and apologized for having to depend on his son to take out the garbage, check the furnace, pay the paper girl, and wash up his dishes. In the evening, the list of tasks included getting the mail for Joe. John noticed that three of the envelopes seemed to indicate that his father's bill payments were overdue, so he asked about the matter. Joe reluctantly admitted that he had not been keeping up with his finances and knew things were a bit "messed up." John offered to help him over the weekend.

On the fourth evening, John was surprised to find his father shaven, cheerful, and much more animated than he had been since long before his fall on the ice. Furthermore, Joe had no tasks in mind for John, but opened a couple of beers and directed his son to sit down. "I've decided to move to Woodsview," he said. "I hate to leave here where your mother and I were happy, but I need to get back into life again." With considerable relief, John complimented Joe on his decision and asked how he could help. The men agreed that John would contact the home's administrator and find a realtor to list the house. Joe wanted to think a bit about how to handle various pieces of his valued sports equipment, although he did not have much concern for what would be done with the furniture and household items. Joe decided to keep his small tent and some basic camping gear, but he sold or gave away his guns. Given his hearing loss and the death or illness of many of his hunting friends, Joe finally admitted to himself that he was unlikely to hunt again. He hoped to swim more regularly after the move, but that would not require much equipment.

Within several months after Joe's move to Woodsview, he reduced his weight on the well-balanced meals provided, became a regular member of a walking group at the nearby shopping mall, and was interviewed about his years as a volunteer fireman by a female Woodsview resident, who wrote articles for the weekly neighborhood newspaper.

John and his family visited every weekend, and some friend or relative usually stopped in midweek. They often found that Joe was either out somewhere or playing cards in the Woodsview living room. He made new friends of both sexes, and his family knew that Joe's good humor had returned when he quoted another octogenarian saying, "My doctors have forbidden me to chase women unless they are going downhill."

Although life in general was certainly better for Joe, his confusion about finances increased, so John offered to manage them for him. They learned from an attorney that Joe could keep control while giving John the authority he needed to help by using a Durable Power of Attorney. Joe asked a number of questions about what John was doing at first and continued over several months to write his own checks and then would forget to record them. It spite of the imperfect system, Joe was visibly relieved to have this general responsibility on his son's shoulders rather than his.

The following January, Joe called John to say he was leaving for three days to go cross-country skiing with friends from his walking group. John was rather alarmed to learn that Joe had traded his tent and camping equipment for cross-country skis, boots, and poles, since he didn't think his father had ever done Nordic skiing before. Joe assured his son that he had, indeed, done so as a young man and that this was a special trip for senior citizens, so it included lessons. John started to tell Joe that he could get killed, then decided it was a foolish comment to make to an almost 84-year-old man.

Maybe it was "better to die with your boots on," even ski boots. Keeping up with his father now that he had moved to Assisted Living was going to be a new type of challenge! John felt "older" than his father and wondered if he, rather than Joe, might be the person needing assistance.

PETER AND RUTH HEREUX

Analytical readers aware of the complex conditions facing octogenarians, Ruth and Peter Hereux, can easily make a list of concrete actions they should take to address their numerous medical, household and financial management, and social support system needs. Intuitive or emotional readers would undoubtedly declare that someone should step right in and help this obviously needful, elderly couple. Yet, those who have dealt with close friends or relatives in similar circumstances will see the possible pitfalls in either expecting Peter and Ruth to logically solve their own problems or arranging for someone else to take charge of their lives.

Like other persons in one of life's final scenes, Peter and Ruth have experienced numerous losses and are being confronted with questions about their own ultimate worth and concerns about the imminence of death. Still, neither is fully aware of the extent of even their physical deficits, let alone their spiritual or social ones. Elderly persons tend to blame one condition, such as loss of hearing or eyesight, for the dependent situation in which they find themselves. Yet, for most elderly people, the greatest problems caused by physical changes result from the multiple effects of life's losses on the aging person's self-concept and relations with others. In addition, each additional loss becomes a reminder of the ongoing aging process and may predict even more losses and death.

In spite of loving and persistent efforts, neither neighbors nor family members could get Peter and Ruth to look at their current situation in its entirety. One or the other would occasionally indicate concern about a problem the other was having. Even less often, Peter or Ruth would admit to some failing on his or her own part, such as forgetfulness or lack of energy to complete a task. It seemed impossible to have a substantive discussion with the two of them together. Nevertheless, since neither seemed to have any time or activities apart from the other, it was almost impossible for those concerned to have a frank, private conversation with either Peter or Ruth.

Peter's son Harold and the Ruth's daughter Ann seemed to be the most determined to help the elderly couple identify the nature and extent of the issues which needed to be handled. Both alternated between gentle coaxing and open confrontation, never certain what emotional or action response they might get as a result. Although Peter was generally gracious in thanking others for their help, he increasingly lapsed into periods of intense anger. Peter seemed to feel that his dependence on others because of his physical problems made him less valued as a man. During these times, he reminded Ruth, his children, and any friends who offered help and advice that he had achieved "the good life" by his own efforts and that he was still making the decisions.

Ruth was likely to agree with whomever was physically present and then contradict herself in the next conversation. Efforts of relatives and friends to get her to realize that she and Peter needed to make decisions only prompted her standard response, "We're doing the best we can." No one disagreed with that, but some were convinced that the best was no longer adequate to protect either the safety or the quality of Peter's and Ruth's lives.

It was not until Peter developed pneumonia and was hospitalized that the scene changed. The several days while her husband was hospitalized were, of course, very difficult for Ruth. She realized she had always assumed Peter would die first, since that had been the experience of so many of her friends. Still, she had never permitted herself to think about how her daily life would change after Peter's death. Now, she began to consider what she would do.

Ruth did not fear her own death. Most of her friends were now gone and she felt that there was nothing else she truly wanted to do. Her family and her home were always central to her life, and she now found both of them larger and more confusing than she really liked. Why, she could not even begin to name all of her great-grandchildren and had difficulty remembering where her grandchildren lived and to whom they were married, or if they still were married. As far as her household was concerned, she seemed to have trouble finding the simplest things and had forgotten she had ever owned many of her once valued possessions.

While Peter was ill, Ruth concluded that it was time for her to decide what she did value at her age and get rid of everything else as soon as she could. Ruth knew she was the type of person who did not want to be alone, so she had decided long ago that she would not remain in her home without Peter. Instead, she expected to move to some type of home with other elderly people and cheerful staff to help her in her final years.

After Peter returned home from the hospital, his daughter Jane came out to spend a week helping care for him. Realizing that her father seemed ready to accept the possibility that additional illness and even death could occur in the near future, she arranged for her father's attorney to stop by to discuss his affairs and make sure his plans were in order. While Ruth was noticeably uneasy about this discussion, she was pleasant and cooperative. On a second visit, the attorney brought copies of a Living Will, a Durable Power of Attorney for Financial Affairs, and a Medical Power of Attorney. He explained each of these to Peter, and discussed with him who would be most appropriate to handle the financial and the medical powers. Peter decided that Ruth, as his wife, should have the Medical Power of Attorney, since none of his children were located nearby. He named his daughter to succeed Ruth. Peter asked his older son to take responsibility for handling his individual financial affairs with his younger son as the back-up. Jane mentioned to Ruth's daughter, Ann, that Peter had taken these steps and that they might want to support Ruth in taking similar actions. Since she had found her father quite willing to take these planning steps, Jane again brought up the subject of Peter's and Ruth's interest in moving to a retirement home of some type. They agreed to let her investigate local options, indicating that they might like an apartment with nursing care nearby, but that they were not willing to go to a nursing home. Peter was especially insistent that he did not want to be where others would tell him what to do. Ruth seemed more concerned about giving up their privacy and changing her surroundings, even though she had already decided she would move if something happened to Peter.

The home scene after Peter's pneumonia hospitalization appeared to be like the previous one; however, it was not nearly as happy or comfortable. In fact, visitors felt that both Peter and Ruth were just hanging by a thread to their independent lives. Throughout the next several months, neither Peter nor Ruth went out much and few people came to see them, saying that they hesitated to interrupt their rest or privacy. When Ruth's daughter, Ann, arrived for a visit several months after the surgery, she found both of them trying desperately to follow a daily routine, but with little energy or interest to motivate their activities. It appeared that rising and dressing, getting some type of food on the table, cleaning up the dishes, and answering occasional telephone calls from family members or neighbors were all that either could accomplish.

Each day of her visit seemed to Ann to be more dreary than the previous one. Knowing that Jane had completed her information gathering about local retirement homes, she asked about their plans at this point. Ruth seemed willing to consider the possibilities, but Peter would not even discuss the matter saying only that they would decide when they were ready.

With frequent visits from family members, numerous telephone updates between Peter and Ruth's children and their parents' physicians, and whatever personal method of keeping calm each concerned person used, they all managed to live through almost four months of improvising, for lack of a script updated to fit the main characters. Suddenly Peter fell, fractured his leg, and had to be hospitalized. He seemed bewildered and upset to find himself in the hospital. But as much as he hated it, he regarded the hospital as a place to get well. So Peter was extremely angry to be moved to a nursing home within a week after his fall, declaring that he was not "crazy" like the other residents there. He insisted he should be at home if he no longer needed hospital care.

Even after he gained strength, Peter continued to blame the family members whom he held responsible for his nursing home placement, including his wife. Initially, friends and children brought Ruth to see him often. Although he was depressed when she did not come, he seldom had much to say to her when she did visit. He talked mostly about what he had once accomplished in business and how others failed to appreciate his efforts. Ruth invariably left discouraged and saddened by her husband's barrage of complaints. She often thought about the words of John Barrymore, "A man is not old until regrets take the place of dreams." Fortunately, Peter gradually became accustomed to the daily routine in the home and seemed somewhat content, if not happy, to be cared for. Unfortunately, he never seemed fully able to recover his sense of time and place following his fall and fracture.

It appeared that Ruth and Peter would live through their next scenes in separate surroundings because of their different needs and responses to life at this point. Ruth's children helped her to decide what she would do after it became apparent that Peter would have to stay in the nursing home. Ruth insisted she wanted to be close to her old neighborhood, in a pretty place with friendly people. While she would like to have a big room, with a good window for plants, that concern seemed secondary to the others. Since Ruth did not need total care, her children soon found a residence for elderly women that was located in a lovely, old mansion in Ruth's lifelong Ohio community and appeared to meet their mother's list of priorities. It even offered a large southern window! The Hereux house was temporarily rented, since Peter refused to sell.

Ruth took very few items with her—photograph albums and loose photos to arrange for a "picture wall," several books of familiar poetry, her favorite yellow- and blue-hued "practical" clothes, jewelry Peter had given her for special anniversaries, several flowering plants, and a few pieces of furniture and decorative objects. Ruth gave away most of her "dress-up" clothes, costume jewelry, and household items, to the delight of her grandchildren and great-grandchildren.

Ruth was a joy to visit in her new home. She did not go out often and found it increasingly difficult to read or do any craft work. Still, she was serene and loving and often commented "I've had a happy life." While she seemed at peace with herself and was not often involved in activities, she appeared to enjoy hearing what others were doing. She sometimes tried to talk with Peter by telephone, but never asked to visit him. Sharing meals and watching TV in the living room with the other residents were especially pleasant times for Ruth. Once when a young visitor asked her if there was enough to keep her busy, Ruth read her the words of C.J. Newman, "The charm of age, my dear, is not to stage a desperate rebellion against what needs to be, but to be."

She carefully followed human interest stories on TV and occasionally became very agitated about news developments that concerned her. A few well-meaning staff and friends tried to convince Ruth that she didn't need to concern herself with such matters. Nevertheless, she wrote letters to the editor of the local newspaper and even kept up her lifelong practice of sending birthday notes to friends and family members.

Many who had never met Ruth were warmed and amused by her caring letters, as were family and friends who received her wonderful birthday notes. Likewise, staff members and residents of the home were often personally told by Ruth how much she loved them. Ruth's graceful acceptance of necessary assistance in advanced age gave her an admirable dignity. Whatever you call it, all agreed that knowing Ruth Hereux in this scene of her life was a real privilege.

Taking Control Strategies For Transitions

CHAPTER SIX

"I am myself at this age. It took me all these years to put the missing pieces together, to confront my own age in terms of integrity and generativity, moving into the unknown future with a comfort now, instead of being stuck in the past. I have never felt so free."

—BETTY FRIEDAN

SUCCESS OR FAILURE IN TRANSITION CONTROL

Having read about the changes experienced by our characters at critical junctures in their lives, let us consider what we can learn from their examples. This chapter explains through examination of the lives of these typical men and women some common strategies that can be effective in dealing with transitions during our aging years. Numerous materials are available to guide us in specific types of planning tasks. This book does not include either the definitive guidelines or detailed information required for completing tasks such as selecting housing, managing finances, or deal-ing with health issues. Be sure to use current information and objective materials as a basis for planning rather than sales pieces provided by a single company or organization that stands to benefit from your decision. This chapter offers general principles for handling these issues as well as examples of planning strategies applied to some typical situations faced by aging persons.

I hope you noted as you read which people seemed to plan effectively and how they decided on their next scenes. Unfortunately, we do not need characters in a book to help us think of men or women whose lives have become increasingly tragic as they moved through Act III. We prob-ably all know people who appear to have made poor deci-sions as they aged. These women or men either failed to recognize the normalcy of changes, neglected to plan before starting a new scene, or did not plan well.

In my estimation, the Endicotts, the Stines, Bessie Smith, Joe Swenson, and Ruth Hereux have planned reasonably well for their next scenes within the possibilities available to them. Like most of us, none has planned flawlessly. The Endicotts have not answered all of the questions they need to; still, both have compromised, and they have committed themselves to make further plans. The Stines had not fully considered their mutual priorities and options before their move after Larry's retirement, although they could not have known that Sybil would have a stroke. Yet, they seem now to be starting a happier and more realistic scene for both of them. Bessie Smith certainly has regrets and a deep sense of loss, but she has moved into a new life role where she is once again reaching out to others. Joe Swenson balked about getting help for awhile, but has now willingly turned over some of his tasks to either his son or his care providers in exchange for greater peace of mind and some new activities. Sadly, Peter Hereux probably never will come to terms with either his memory losses or his physical condition. Yet, Ruth has turned her life around, is accepting care from others, and is radiating warmth and love to those around her.

Jerry and Maria Rodriguez appear to be in the midst of a very unpleasant scene without a clear way to end it and start a better one. While there are a number of difficult issues here, the key reasons for the failure of their plan to move to Florida are that the plan was not a mutual one and that neither Jerry nor Maria took sufficient time to work through their various concerns. Olivia Wilson's children approached planning for their mother's next scene with appropriate reason and concern. Since we know that Olivia has made other transitions in her life rather effectively, the main problem this time appears to be that she does not feel she made her own final choice to move into her Continuing Care Retirement Community. This type of facility seems to be very suitable for Olivia in this scene of her life, but she must feel accepted and wanted in this place, or she may never be happy here. Of course, we cannot know for sure whether she would feel better about the atmosphere if she had a sense of ownership about the decision. It is not uncommon for elderly persons to make a firm decision and, later, forget how and why they did so. These situations are painfully difficult for family members and friends to bear. Nevertheless, loved ones can feel more comfortable with the results, knowing they did all they could to support the aging persons, in making their own decisions.

HELPING OTHERS MAKE THIRD ACT DECISIONS

Friends, family members, and professionals who assist older people in deciding how to live through the diverse scenes in Act III need to have an understanding of the aging process, good helping skills, and knowledge about dealing with transitions. It is important to be honestly open and as unbiased as possible during this helping process. The person facing change should reconsider or evaluate the type of transition he or she is experiencing, make a realistic appraisal of the situation, develop a new script using appropriate information and move toward a new beginning.

Most of us find it difficult to understand a situation when we are in the midst of it, as the old saying about not being able to see the forest for the trees reminds us. Consequently, we fail to realize how much time and effort it will take to adjust and redirect our lives. We may doubt or blame ourselves for not handling things well, although the main impetus for change may be outside our control—as local economic conditions, family relations, or certain health factors often are. Older women and men tend to isolate themselves and feel embarrassed about not handling things well even more than younger people do.

Adult children who cannot put aside their own fears of illness and death or see beyond their personal interests in how a parent's assets are used can do more harm than good, just as Olivia Wilson's overbearing son-in-law did. In these cases, loving family members would do well to encourage their parents to rely on either capable friends or qualified counselors to assist them in their planning and, then, stay out of the way. Most mentally competent aging parents do try to consider the possible affects of their decisions on other family members. In today's world, where both husbands and wives often work full time and live many miles away, aging parents should not make crisis management of their issues become a way of life for either concerned neighbors, friends, or family members.

RECYLING YOUR STRATEGIES
FOR CREATING NEW SCRIPTS

People facing changes certainly benefit by having others with whom to share their concerns. They also need a cognitive framework for dealing not only with the issues they face, but also with their feelings about losing control over their lives. Few of us reach age 50 without knowing what it is like to feel "trapped, up against a brick wall, or stymied," even though we may also have experienced many periods of relative stability. In reaction to these feelings of frustration, we have either "muddled through" or used some type of planning, problem-solving, or decision-making process. Some of us are deliberate and aware of the process we normally use to face problems. Others seem to be casual, even "laid back." Few of us would want to eliminate the possibility of serendipity, some unexpected joy or opportunity.

Still, almost all of those who make sound decisions either have "in their heads" or "on paper" several steps or guidelines they depend on which they have developed through personal experience. For example, you may have laughed the first time your mother told you not to go to sleep angry with someone, and you hated having your father insist that you fix a mistake before quitting when you were tired. Yet, you may have taught your children the same principles and followed them yourself all of your adult life.

Whether or not you have been aware of certain problem-solving or decision-making patterns in your own life, I urge you now to stop and consider what steps or guidelines have usually worked for you—and what approaches did not. In a way, the strategies you employ become part of your plot line for your current scene and lead into the next one. This chapter presents eight strategies for taking control during transitions. These strategies are explained in subsequent pages and presented graphically in Figure 6.1.

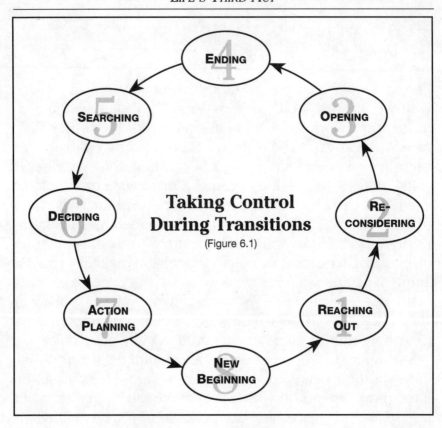

It is important to note that each person's life drama includes a series of transition cycles leading to new challenges and commitments. Nevertheless, the methods we use to maintain personal control are essentially the same throughout our performances, so in a sense, we recycle or reuse strategies that worked for us. Figure 6.2 illustrates this repetition of the planning process.

My terms for these transition control strategies are:

1. Reaching out	5. Searching
2. Reconsidering	6. Deciding
3. Opening	7. Action planning
4. Ending	8. New beginning

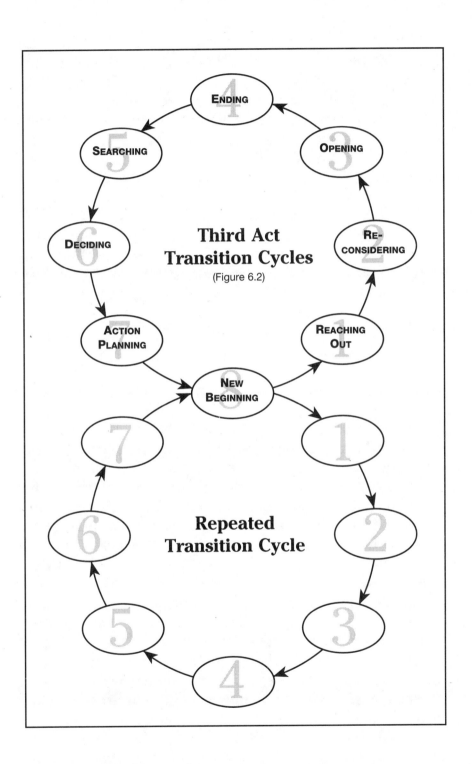

Third Act Transition Cycles
(Figure 6.2)

ENDING 4

SEARCHING 5

OPENING 3

DECIDING 6

RE-CONSIDERING 2

ACTION PLANNING 7

REACHING OUT 1

NEW BEGINNING 8

Repeated Transition Cycle

You might ask, why is the "beginning" at the end? The beginning of a new scene is not the first step in transition planning, but the result of using the preliminary strategies. These strategies are useful repeatedly throughout life as we move toward new scenes. New beginnings, which must follow an ending, are typically full of promise and excitement. More often than not, during the early part of a new scene, our lives seem to go smoothly. We manage both our daily tasks and even the most challenging, unfamiliar tasks capably. Generally, as we begin a new scene, we are in control. Because we feel in control, even if a bit nervous about our new roles, many of us become optimistic and invigorated at these times. We are also usually able to relate well to others who are part of our lives.

REACHING OUT

Reaching out happens after the new scene is underway and describes how people extend themselves to consider the concerns of others and, in some cases, reach out to help them. The time during which Bessie Smith served as the self-appointed counselor of members of her church was such a period. As long as you remain reasonably healthy, both physically and emotionally, this scene and others with similar scripts filled with enjoying, helping, and caring can last for many years with only minor lifestyle changes. These mini-transitions to similar but new scenes will be prompted every few months or years, either by our own developing interests or by new opportunities.

Some mini-transitions will be initiated by losses rather than opportunities. Often, these are not totally negative experiences, although they may involve replacing a previously enjoyed activity or relationship with a new activity or friendship group. For example, gaining more time to play golf may make giving up competitive, singles tennis tolerable. Or, having a friend or spouse offer to take a daily exercise walk with you may be an excellent reason to give up jogging. Another example common to aging women and men is becoming well acquainted or reacquainted with another person, while sharing in the illness or death of a mutual friend. Even times of grieving may present opportunities for renewing ties with family members with whom you were too busy to keep in close touch during your active employment and parenting years.

RECONSIDERING

We can generally make minor adjustments to our lives for some time during our Third Act. Then, it seems that a number of things invariably start to go wrong. Eventually, more major challenges occur that force us to reconsider the way we currently live. Sometimes the challenge is sudden and dramatic, whether the change happens directly to you or to someone close to you. More typically, the changes occur gradually in the form of deficits or losses. Normal physical changes occur in our hearing, seeing, tasting, smelling, short-term memory, reaction time, sensitivity to temperature change, sense of balance, muscular strength, bone mass, and sexual capacity or responsiveness.

Significant or multiple changes in the conditions amid which we live also affect us. These include retiring from our jobs, medical problems, the death or moving away of those on whom we have depended, and giving up our homes. Less personal losses, but potentially powerful ones, are changes in community life, healthcare, communications, politics, or technology. Since these external conditions do not all change at once, we typically ignore such changes until we are forced by circumstances to confront the reality of their impact on us. Then, we occasionally feel overwhelmed by our sense of being out of control or thrust into an unfamiliar scene. Like Olivia Wilson, alone in her apartment, some people retreat to familiar surroundings and stop trying to relate to the rest of society.

Most aging people cope effectively with these gradual changes, and usually, with the sudden ones as well. In cases of gradual change, older people either know friends who have similar conditions, they expected such losses, or they have other positive life conditions. Nevertheless, numerous or sudden changes in health, fears of being alone or unable to access necessary services, continuing depression, or a rapid drop in your standard of living can make coping very difficult.

When we confront major challenges or feel overwhelmed by a series of minor ones, our "basic training" may serve us poorly. Many of us were taught to "stick with it," "hang in there," "keep our noses to the grindstone," or "keep up a brave front." Consequently, as we near the end of a current life scene or cycle, we may dismiss our strong feelings of dissatisfaction or fail to admit increasing difficulty with activities we once either enjoyed or did well. Jerry Rodriguez's reaction to his heart attack presents a typical example of one who has trouble in changing his lifestyle. Initially, the pleasure he finds in writing his stories and sharing them with his grandchildren helps him to partially accept the loss of his daily work roles.

Instead of ignoring the signals, persistent shouts of "scene change" from the stage hands should lead us to reconsider and to focus on the apparent source of the problem, in preparation for making a positive transition. Our characters didn't change their lives by just cheerfully announcing that it was now time to plan a new scene. Instead, they agonized, argued, and avoided until, finally, they seemed to have no choices but to deal with their situations. We probably behave in much the same way.

As you make yourself reconsider your situation, put your

first emphasis on getting the problem issues identified. You need to ask yourself questions like,

1. What's actually going on here?
2. Is this an expected transition?
3. Did I bring this on, or did my spouse, my children, or my society change somehow?
4. How is this affecting me—my relationships, routines, roles, and thinking?
5. Is this a temporary or a permanent change?
6. Have I identified the basic problem area, or just some symptoms?
7. Are there, in fact, several changes happening at once?

Once you identify the nature of your primary challenge—a financial, medical, or housing change, for example—you are ready to open yourself to new possibilities.

OPENING

At this point in a life scene, you have not necessarily decided to develop a new script and begin your next scene. You are merely agreeing to be open to the possibility of doing so if you decide to end the current scene. Now that you have identified the basic challenge or set of challenges, you should provide your own honest answers to these additional questions:

1. Does the loss or change really matter?
2. Does it imply more serious changes?
3. How am I coping with the situation?
4. Am I declining or developing?
5. Why is this change affecting me this way?

In cases of major loss, such as the death of a spouse or a major physical change in either you or your partner, some of the answers are obvious to most of us. For example,

Olivia Wilson realized that she faced a new life after her husband's death, but she had considerable difficulty recognizing the impact of gradual changes in her health and social relationships over the years.

Does The Loss Or Change Really Matter?
Does It Imply More Serious Changes?

Our responses to gradual or smaller losses vary considerably. You may find losing your sense of taste or smell annoying, but not really troublesome in comparison with losing your ability to quickly adapt to changing light conditions. To you, driving under all conditions may be more important than enjoying the subtleties of gourmet cooking. A man who has lived alone may easily move to a new residence with fewer household responsibilities, while a woman living alone finds it extremely difficult to give up her own home. Like the actress who has long played romantic leads, but is now invited to act the part of the ingenue's mother, we strongly resist giving up the roles that have defined how we regard ourselves or seem to be essential to our sense of personal independence. You can probably think of specific losses that would disturb you, but would not bother your best friend.

How Am I Coping With The Situation?

Your main task at this stage of planning is to know your own attitudes toward others and yourself. You need to know—and frequently remind yourself—that effective living in our mature years is based on both healthy attitudes and good decision-making skills. Aging is not the opposite of growth, but a normal part of the adult development process. Your Third Act can be the exciting and fulfilling culmination of a developmental span that has been continuous from conception rather than a gloomy period of decline from the peak of the good life. True, certain occurrences tend to be associated with advanced age just as other unpleasant occurrences are normal in early childhood, teenage, or middle years. Like puberty, aging is a natural and inevitable process, not the equivalent to being incompetent or sick.

Am I Declining Or Developing As I Age?

We tend to define "old" in various ways, depending on our point of view. In terms of chronological age, "old" often means being 65 or more, being retired, or being eligible for social security. Old is also defined according to the physical characteristics of posture, hair color, facial features, agility, and abilities to hear and see. Old suggests certain behavioral characteristics—slow reaction time, altering sleeping or urination patterns, rigidity of ideas or opinions, forgetfulness, resistance to change, and irritability—even though many aging people do not have all of those problems. Certain social roles imply age: grandparent, retiree, or resident of a special place.

Old is increasingly defined by self-report—how we regard ourselves. While aging is not just a "state of mind," aging is certainly affected by one's state of mind. The person who finds meaning in life through involvement in some valued activity or loving relationship is more apt to solve a problem or work around it than one who has lost interest in living. Your perceptions of your role as an aging person not only reflect reality, but also create reality.

Why Is This Change Affecting Me In This Way?

Some people have lifetime patterns of living that make it easier for them to adapt to aging than for others. People who generally have been optimistic and have established patterns of serving others have more positive self-concepts than do those whose lives have been marked by a lack of warm relationships with their parents or the death of a sibling or parent during their childhood. Women or men who regard themselves negatively typically have to work harder to deal with aging and may require more professional assistance than others do as they make new plans. Persons who have been flexible in their thinking can adapt to the challenges of aging better than those who have been rigid. Being flexible implies enjoying surprises, being accepting of diverse values and opinions, trying new things, and having strong emotions. People who are rigid insist on familiar surroundings and routines and feel little need for new experiences or learning.

ENDING

No, I am not talking about the ending of life! We are still discussing transition planning strategies—taking and keeping control during periods of change in your life. Once you are certain that you face a significant challenge that will prevent you from living as you have been, or you recognize that you have become quite dissatisfied with the current state of your life, it's time to take the next step, which I call ending. The time has come to end your current scene. This means stopping some of what you have been doing and figuring out how best to live well in the next scene of your life. Take Sybil and Larry Stine as examples. In their situation, they faced a major medical challenge and a series of smaller issues or dissatisfactions with their lives.

Sybil's stroke and her physical debilities presented major challenges to both of them. Their growing financial concerns and the uncertainties about Larry's prostate condition were also rather significant issues. In addition, their mutual, but previously unshared dissatisfactions with the retirement lifestyle of cocktail parties and rather superficial social relations, as well as their loss of a place to garden, were also motivations for making a scene change. You will recall that shortly after Sybil's hospitalization, they remodeled their retirement home to accommodate Sybil's physical limitations. However, in order to deal effectively with the remaining issues, they have to be willing to completely end the scene they chose at retirement and to script a new one.

Their decision, after considering various alternatives, is to move to another community and to emphasize a different set of activities. We can imagine that it will be awkward for them to tell long-time friends of this change, fearing perhaps that others will regard them as emotionally unstable or in great financial difficulty. Still, they face their changes openly and recognize that they do not want to continue as they have been living and do not need to stay in the retirement setting that they originally selected.

Like the Stines, each of us occasionally must find the personal courage to end what we either no longer wish to do, or cannot do, before we are ready to imagine alternative scripts for the next scene. Such courage may be required at several junctures throughout the Third Act. Remember that these are not failures, but result from normal conditions or developments for adults. We first give up childish things in order to become adults, and, in some ways, we have been giving up in order to make new gains ever since. As we move through life, we give up some of our beliefs, our attachments to others, our dreams for our children and ourselves, and our valued possessions. We replace them with others. This is inevitably painful and difficult. By letting go we have grown. In the same manner, we are capable of continuing to grow and change until death.

SEARCHING

Once you have made a decision to end a previous scene, you are probably not yet completely prepared to plan a new script. This time in your planning is one of searching. To others, this may look like you are continuing to play out the previous scene as you go through the motions of your life. Only you, and those closest to you, will realize that you are tackling the essential task of determining the next focus or purpose of your life. Making personal decisions can be more difficult than making business or academic decisions, primarily because we first need to decide on our purpose or new goal. No one else can tell you what will give your life direction and meaning.

Some people do their searching almost entirely alone, usually testing their thinking with one or more trusted people before they move ahead to the decision stage. If you really know yourself well and have learned to formulate and clarify problem situations, searching in solitude can be very effective. This may include reading of motivational and informational material. For some, it will also involve prayer, meditation, and, perhaps, retreat to a different setting for awhile. When we are deciding on a new purpose or focus in our lives largely by ourselves we still have to be bold enough to test our ideas with a few other trusted persons. And, we need to be open to reexamining our thinking if those who know us well regard the proposed commitment as unrealistic.

On the other hand, if you're a person who usually benefits from sharing ideas with others at each stage of your thinking, you may wish to involve friends, family members, and professionals at an early point in your searching. This is certainly advisable if you are feeling quite depressed by your recent losses and believe your present life has little meaning or value. It is also necessary when the problem you face is very complex or you lack sufficient information about the conditions which are forcing changes in your life, whether those conditions are medical, financial, psychological, or environmental. While loved ones can be helpful, professional counselors are normally more objective and have training in how to guide your thinking without deciding for you. A counselor may enable you to get excellent insights on your situation and provide accurate information, sometimes at little or no charge to people who do not require extensive amounts of time or individually customized data. When there is considerable cost involved, your insurance coverage may be limited to half of the cost of counseling for a limited number of visits, but other community resources may be available to pay for the remainder, if you are unable to do so.

Your community Area Agency for the Aging can provide information and also direct you to another agency, such as legal assistance or home healthcare, which offers the specific assistance you seek. Your physician or Health Maintenance Organization (HMO), a rabbi or pastor, your bank officer, a senior citizen's center staff member, or the admissions director for a nearby residence for the aging will often be happy to schedule an appointment to talk about your concerns and your ideas for emphasis in the next stage of your life. Active friends, community counselors, and others who seem to live full and satisfying lives may also be good resources for you. Most people are flattered to have you ask for their help and will appreciate the fact that you have your searching task clearly identified.

As we recall our characters, note that Maria Rodriguez made a decision about where she and her husband should move based on the advice of just one other person; however, she is certainly not an example of a person who uses searching to clarify a new purpose or who relies on an experienced and objective person with whom to test her ideas. On the contrary, she appears to skip the searching process entirely and makes a decision without considering either Jerry's interests or other alternatives. Joe Swenson, probably not an analytical type, nevertheless does take some time alone after his hospitalization to reconsider and clarify what is important to him. Using information that his son has helped him acquire, he finally makes his solitary decision to leave his home and to develop some new interests.

As you discuss your situation with other people, be sure to clarify that you are seeking self-understanding and information about a possible new emphasis for your life at this time, not specific recommendations for action. You are still searching for your new purpose and are not quite ready to decide precisely what you are going to do and how you are going to accomplish it. It is too soon to consider alternative action plans, and you certainly do not want anyone telling you what to do. You want good listeners and questioners, not directions. You may want to leave the door open to return for more reactions and ideas from people you find helpful when you are ready to consider how to achieve the goal you select.

While it is useful to think of these steps to beginning a new life scene as sequential, in real life we usually combine some of the steps and also retrace our steps until we get on the right path. For example, you may be searching for your new focus while you develop and compare new alternative scripts. By imagining yourself acting out a possible script you may realize how uncomfortable or how exciting a specific new purpose for your life could be, therefore helping to clarify your next scene's major emphasis.

DECIDING

Now that you have taken the preliminary steps towards reconsidering your present situation, opening yourself to changing the script, preparing to end your current scene, and searching for a new life emphasis, you are finally ready to start on the decision-making part of your transition.

Precisely how you handle decisions depends on both the

situation in which you find yourself and on your personality. People have varying degrees of tolerance for ambiguity; some can comfortably go a long while without definite answers to critical questions while others are eager to get almost any decision made, just so matters will be clear. Your self-concept can also affect how you make decisions. If you lack confidence in your decision-making skills—or in your own capability to carry out your decisions—you may become overly anxious about what others believe you should do. As a consequence, you may move too quickly to satisfy those people rather than dealing fully with your own deepest needs.

Your beliefs about control also influence how you make decisions. People who emphasize self-control tend to believe that their lives are primarily the result of their own behavior. They are likely to believe that their personal choices of action lead to their future rewards and risks. On the other hand, those who emphasize external factors believe that what happens to us is largely determined by other people or by "fate." Obviously, one who emphasizes self-control is more apt to do the work necessary to collect information and to evaluate the alternatives for action than the man or woman who regards events as largely beyond individual control.

A final personality trait that influences your decisions is how willing you are to take risks. Some people appear to thrive on risky situations, while others try to avoid risk at all costs. Today, we may have real difficulties with determining what risk actually is. For example, financial advisors have often recommended that young and middle-aged adults take risks with significant proportions of their investments and that older adults be more conservative. Yet, increasingly advisors urge even retired persons to keep major percentages of their assets in equity investments, once regarded as relatively high risk, pointing out that not to do so results in the risk of "out-living your money." And, in the area of lifestyle, mature adults have traditionally been expected to "slow down" and to take fewer physical risks. Yet, we now know that strenuous exercise may actually prolong life for some and can certainly improve the quality of life for most of us. My retired friend, Al, who recently bicycled across the United States raising funds for Alzheimer's research a year after surgery for prostate cancer is one of many examples. Maybe it is risky not to take risks as we age!

You need to know both yourself and your situation very well before moving ahead to make decisions. Deciding always requires a series of steps, whether you face a major decision or a small one. The following five steps are critical to decision-making when you face a transition:

1. Reaffirm your new purpose or life role
2. Identify possible alternatives
3. Compare these alternatives
4. Test the preferred alternatives
5. Select one alternative

Reaffirm Your New Purpose Or Life Role

The first task in creating a new life scene is to be absolutely certain you have defined a clear purpose or focus for the next phase of your life. This implies you also have decided which parts of your role in the previous scene will change. If you are making a scene change involving another person, such as your spouse or housemate, that person's role changes and personality also need to be considered in adopting your purpose or focus for the next scene. Among our characters, the Endicotts and the Stines are good examples of couples who worked carefully through their differences by developing both mutual and individual purposes and priorities. By contrast, Maria Rodriguez largely ignored

Jerry's needs in her eagerness to get to Florida, with negative results for both of them. Olivia Wilson's son-in-law was so eager to get her new financial and housing arrangements settled that he and her children neglected to fully consider Olivia's personality and interests.

Identify Possible Alternatives

The second decision task of identifying possible alternatives may take some time, especially when the next scene is expected to require a major scene change. James Endicott, probably wisely, deferred to Sarah's resistance to making a major shift in location, getting an agreement from her to reconsider that issue annually and to gather information about other settings in the meantime. Although James made the major change to retirement, he and Sarah developed an alternative scenario that required his wife to make only minor changes in her work and volunteer roles during the same scene.

In cases where people are either physically or emotionally disabled or lack skills in collecting information about alternative options—often when they become quite elderly—either family members or professional advisors will need to help with the tasks of developing alternatives. Neither Joe Swenson nor Ruth Hereux was able to independently research the necessary data about possible Assisted Living homes. Nevertheless, both were happy with the results and felt that they were in control of the decisions. No doubt, this is because Joe and Ruth were assisted by their respective adult children and professionals who lovingly considered what was most important to them at this stage of life. Note also that people concerned about Joe and Ruth made every effort to get them to understand the alternatives and to make their own decisions. The Stines had some big issues with which to deal, so they were very methodical about the way in which they talked through both the obvious and the more hidden concerns for each of them and developed a list of alternatives. They also spent several months sharing the tasks of collecting detailed information after they decided which alternatives were worth further consideration.

Most of us need encouragement to imagine or dream a little wider than our Third Act minds—long burdened with responsibilities and concerns—have allowed us to do since our early adult years. Do not ignore or throw out attractive alternatives too rapidly. Larry and Sybil Stine's modified "brainstorming" technique was fun and ultimately productive, primarily because it freed them to share their deepest thoughts and to have to fun. Considering the possibilities of making kites or living on a houseboat may also have made it easier to face making the big decision to turn their backs on their original retirement community and start a new scene in a different community. Do list all of the alternatives suggested for later consideration, however unrealistic they may seem at first.

As you develop action alternatives, your major emphasis may be on either better financial management, appropriate healthcare, a new housing arrangement, more satisfying personal relationships, fulfilling volunteer or paid work, a meaningful spiritual life, or just a better pattern and balance for daily living. After you identify the aspects of your life in which you plan to make some improvements, list them in priority order. Our priorities, or dominant needs, change as the scenes of our lives progress. It is imperative that our highest priorities be met as well as possible if we are to feel in control. Olivia Wilson's move to a CCRC addressed her needs for better financial, healthcare, and housing arrangements, but it certainly did not satisfy her social relationship needs or provide her with a happy daily life. Maria Rodriguez shed her work responsibilities and moved to a new house which she herself had chosen. Still, the changes had a negative impact on her physical well-being as well as on her daily life and personal relationships. In those instances, certain high priority needs had not been met for all concerned.

Compare The Alternatives

By the time you believe you have identified all of the alternative scenarios which would help you to refocus or achieve your new purpose, you will be comparing the alternatives. Keep your eye on your chosen focus or purpose as you proceed. Ask yourself the same set of questions about each alternative:

1. What are the likely long- and short-term consequences of following this plan?
2. What are the possible benefits to me and to those close to me?
3. What the the potential risks?
4. What will I gain by this choice?
5. What am I apt to lose?
6. What options will this alternative scene leave open to me for the following scene when I either must or prefer to move on?
7. What options will this script close off for me and for others?
8. Which scenarios really interest or excite me?
9. Which ones either appear boring or look like someone else's life rather than mine?

Test The Preferred Alternatives

As you answer these questions, you will gradually eliminate the less desirable alternatives leaving a few attractive scenarios or action plans for more careful examination. You may even discover a new possibility to add to your list. Now begin to test the preferred alternatives. You might use simulation, probably what concerned people had in mind for Maria and Jerry Rodriguez in suggesting a long vacation in Florida before they decided to move there permanently. In some cases you cannot actually test the plan, but should take the necessary time to imagine or visualize yourself in another scene, as the Endicotts agreed to do and the Stines also did before moving to new areas. Ruth Hereux seemed to be able to picture herself in a sunny room surrounded by loving care as she made her decision to move to a new home. Testing for many of us also involves getting reactions from others about a projected change. It clearly did for Bessie Smith who talked at length with both her children and her pastor. Some people choose to quantify the alternatives, weighing the relative factors involved in their choice. A few will use decision aids which they have used in their work, while others will not find these aids easily applicable to personal planning.

In making your decisions, it is imperative to consider all of the likely positive and negative consequences, benefits and risks. Since "this is your life," it is also critical to know your own feelings and preferences as you select a new role for yourself and move toward developing a new script.

Select One Of The Alternatives

Having identified and compared all of the realistic alternatives, you are ready for the last transition decision-making step—selecting your preferred alternative. Now you are actually deciding. If you have done your homework well, you will select the scene and role that offer the most positive consequences and benefits at the least possible risk to both you and those you love. Ideally, your choice should also leave you with the most attractive options whenever this scene concludes.

Your choice needs to feel comfortable for you—consistent with the person you are. Hopefully, your choice will make it possible for you, like Bessie Smith and Ruth Hereux, to give yourself credit for the life you have led so far rather than leaving you full of regret. Not everyone is so fortunate. During my years in New York City private banking, I met elderly women and men far more fortunate in financial and physical health than either Bessie or Ruth, whose choices to stay in scenes they could no longer truly manage left them bitter and angry. In their failure to plan for the time when they could no longer live safely in Manhattan or handle their own business affairs, they often left their adult children bickering among themselves as they attempted to keep their aging parents from either being killed by a speeding taxi or squandering the family's inheritance.

Regrettably, the final scenes for a few of us will be played after we have lost some of our physical and mental capacity to make good decisions. I urge you to think NOW about these possible scenes. Then, discuss them with your partner and children or close friends and discuss which alternative scripts you prefer in such cases. Key challenges for those who are either incapacitated or incompetent revolve around physical care and financial concerns, often within the context of spiritual and relationship issues.

Discuss alternative medical treatment and financial matters—in case you suffer a severe loss in either your mental or physical capacities—with appropriate professional advisors, such as your banker, attorney, religious advisor, and physician. Ask yourself some hard questions:

1. What type of conditions would need to be present before I would agree that someone else should handle my financial affairs?
2. Should I arrange for that now by establishing a trust fund and granting Durable Power of Attorney or conservatorship authority for my financial affairs under stated conditions?

3. How do I feel about prolonging my life in cases of severe impairment?
4. Under what conditions would I grant to another the authority to make decisions about my treatment, including life-support systems and hospital or nursing home placement?
5. To whom would I entrust that responsibility?
6. What type of funeral and burial do I want?

As soon as you have answered one group of questions, take the necessary legal, financial, healthcare, and end of life planning steps to affirm your decisions.

Imagine that you are writing your obituary. This report or summary of your life depends almost entirely on the very personal actions you take rather than on specific steps directed by professional advisors. The ultimate questions for most of us are:

1. How do I hope to be remembered?
2. What do I want my life and death to mean to those closest to me; to society?
3. Will my obituary describe me as I wish to be recalled?
4. If not, what can I change now to make my preferred obituary more likely?

These are powerful questions. You cannot avoid them if you wish to be in control of all of your Third Act.

ACTION PLANNING

You have made your decision. In practice, selecting your preferred alternative and developing a specific action plan often merge into a single strategy or step. In selecting an alternative, you decide to see yourself in a particular way and begin to envision yourself, perhaps even talk about yourself in that new way. For example, when you decide to move from a large house to an apartment, you may begin to think of where you would shop or exercise, how you would furnish your space to include others whom you wish to invite, and the activities that you hope to enjoy alone. Or perhaps you care little about the furnishings, but can hardly wait to free up some of the money that your large house has required in order to take a trip that you have imagined. Other people are eager to be in a new environment, perhaps out of the city in order to be near the waterfront, the desert, or the mountains.

Since few of us choose to improvise entirely, we develop some concrete plans for the first few days or months of our new scenes. Typically, this involves exacting promises from friends and family to visit or to be in close touch so that we will not feel lonely or deserted in this new life. Some transitioning men and women will commit themselves in advance to new volunteer roles, study groups, social groups, or travel plans as part of the next scene. Many desire to establish the basic plot before beginning a new scene. While we want to allow for the unexpected opportunity, we may dread waking up in a new scene without any clue as to how to play our unfamiliar roles!

As you begin to think about your new role, you'll realize that you not only need to outline the script to get started in your new role, but you also need to figure out how to make the transition from the current scene to the next. Occasionally, you will discover as you begin to be specific about what you will have to give up and what you would do in such a new role that the alternative scene you have selected does not appear to be a good choice for you. Consequently, as you move forward with your action planning, you may need to retrace your steps. Of course, you always need to consider how to make the transition smoothly.

Make The Scene Change

In a dramatic performance, a scene change may require a new set or costumes. The actors must learn new lines. Part of this planning was relatively easy for our characters. Most of them successfully made and implemented plans to divide their property with family members. Some also sold their homes and moved themselves and their remaining possessions to new places. A few had to figure out how to adapt to either sudden or gradual physical losses. While their financial resources varied considerably, all had to analyze their situations and revise their life scripts according to the resources available to them. The Endicotts even established future planning dates to keep them faithful to their scene-change agreements.

By the time we become Third Act players, most mature men and women have become skilled in avoiding specific planning. Nevertheless, doing specific planning is our next task. Developing and acting out the scripts to manage primarily technical matters such as housing, work, finances, and medical care are relatively easy compared with accepting our losses and adapting to our changing social or personal relationships. Our attitudes toward the situation may have more significance for the quality of our mature years than the actual reality of the specific losses. Filling the huge gaps of meaning and activity that result from giving up our roles as respected homeowner, valued employee, community leader, needed son or daughter, or responsible parent sometimes demands more skilled script writing than we are capable of managing alone.

You may have the necessary emotional strength, but need support from others in getting the information you require. Another person may have considerable information, but lack the motivation or confidence to move forward to develop a specific plan. Thinking and dreaming about the new scene will not get you there! Nor will it improve the scene you have concluded you need to change.

Retrace Your Steps If Necessary

If you have faithfully followed the recommended steps for transition planning, now is the time to firm up your new purpose or focus. If it no longer seems attractive or compelling to you, go back to the searching phase of your planning and work back up to the decision-making steps. Give yourself credit for recognizing that you were not on the right track. Now may be the time you would benefit from talking over your feelings of being "out of focus" with a trusted friend or professional advisor.

Take as much time as you need to retrace your steps through the searching and deciding steps, once again developing alternatives and testing them. Then, make a new decision about your next role before moving back to the action planning stage. Do not expect inspired choruses and bright lights to tell you that you have finally made the right decision! Few of us should wait for absolute clarity and confidence. Life is too short. As soon as you are reasonably comfortable and, possibly, rather excited about both your chosen purpose and your action plan, it is time to move to the next scene, to make a new beginning.

NEW BEGINNING

As you begin to develop and live in your new role, keep in mind what you have learned about yourself and the world in which you live—all of the financial, medical, housing, work, and recreation priorities in your life. Remember also what you know about your very personal desires for spiritual development, social relationships, and structure or balance as you develop the script for this scene in your Third

Act. New beginnings are often scary and, therefore, may be rather tentative.

As you practice your new role, you become more confident that the activities and environment you decide to emphasize fit you at this time in your life. In most cases, you will also begin to reach out to include others and to help them according to their needs based on your own experience and talents. Your reaching out may lead you to develop a closer personal relationship with one or more individuals, start a career, or participate in a group service project. Eventually, you will become quite skilled and comfortable in your new role. Then, just as you think you are ready to go "on tour" with this production—after several years, or even several months—something you could not have predicted or written into your script may interfere with your chosen scene. This results in a dramatic interruption in your scene.

Dramatic Interruptions

For Sybil and Larry Stine, this interruption was a stroke. For Olivia Wilson, it was her husband's heart attack and resulting death. For some, it might be new opportunities, as early retirement and a new grandchild were for the Endicotts. Sudden or gradual changes in health, like those experienced by Jerry Rodriguez, Bessie Smith, and Joe Swenson may require that you reconsider your life's focus and plan of action. Once again, you have to face the possibility of changing both your scene and your role.

Starting A New Transition Cycle

Life does, indeed, present us with dramatic interruptions that introduce the possibility of significant changes for our lives. Becoming aware of the need for another transition can be discouraging. You know it requires time and energy on your part to work through the strategies for taking control of your life during each personal transition cycle. The first piece of "good news" is that you have survived another scene in the Third Act and are still part of the cast. The second piece is that you know the strategies for managing a personal transition cycle. You are a seasoned actor on life's stage. The years after age 50 need not be a period of decline from the teenage and middle years of life. Instead, these years offer most of us multiple dramatic scenes and transition cycles, each presenting unique opportunities for growth and pleasure—if we take control of them.

Outstanding Performances

CHAPTER SEVEN

*"Life breaks us all, but many
are stronger in the broken places."*

—Ernest Hemingway

In this final chapter, I want to motivate you to take the next steps in planning for life's Third Act. If you are approaching age 50, that means starting to develop your basic plan for this period of your life. For those of you who are already well into life's Third Act roles, the next moves will be to reconsider your situation and create your script for your future scenes.

This chapter offers assistance with these tasks in two ways: First, it introduces some people I admire who are leading extraordinary lives in their Third Act. Unfortunately, I cannot tell you anymore about what will happen next in the lives of the people we met in the earlier chapters. But, some things are certain. All will continue to face transitions. Some will grow and develop beyond their current situations. A few may lose control over their lives or get "stuck" in roles and scenes that no longer fit their needs. Others will soon die. Second, this chapter reviews the themes and principles presented in earlier chapters so you have a short version of how and why to move ahead with your own planning.

ORDINARY ACTORS LIVING
EXTRAORDINARY SCENES

Sir Richard Steele once said, "There are so few who can grow old with a good grace." I do not believe this is true. There are many well-known examples of individuals and groups of older people who accomplish great deeds in their mature years. These include famous artists, philosophers, and political leaders as well as the less-publicized persons who take Elderhostel trips, share their management skills abroad through SCORE, volunteer through RSVP, or organize their own service projects after they retire. Many authors have described such people and their activities.

Over the years, I have known a number of aging women and men, as you may have. I have appreciated the loving grandparenting my children received, the learned teachers who challenged me, and the wisdom of capable, older men and women with whom I have shared professional and community responsibilities. Still, I suppose that when I was younger, I tended to regard many older people as either peripheral or irrelevant to the most important activities of my own life. I was often too busy and preoccupied with parental, work, and community responsibilities to take the time to get know senior neighbors and relatives. There have even been a few men and women whom I avoided or ignored as much as possible because of their frequent criticisms or complaints.

In recent years, as I began contemplating my own aging, and researched and talked with others about their experiences, I found that I was discovering new attitudes toward older people—and toward myself. Recently, it has been my privilege to become acquainted with some of the diverse and delightful people who live in the Northeast Kingdom of Vermont. One need look no further than this rugged, rural community to find remarkable examples of those who take control of their mature years, although not all the people I include in this chapter live there. Those I interviewed would probably agree with Michael E. De Montaigne's observation, "I speak truth, not so much as I would, but as much as I dare; and I dare a little the more, as I grow older."

As I interviewed these special people for this chapter, I longed to extend our conversations in order to gain from the richness of their life experiences. Regrettably, it has been impossible to tell you in a single chapter all that they shared. Since these women and men have permitted me to use their names, it is especially important to caution that these brief summaries are the equivalent of amateur "snapshots" of each person at one point in their lives. While I have made every effort not to impose themes or strategies for controlling their mature years on any of those interviewed, I did listen especially for the key principles by which they live.

Virginia and John Downs are established Vermonters— eager to make new friends and consider diverse perspectives on a wide range of issues. Now 69 and 74, the Downs have been married 40 years and have four grown children. John, a Yale Law School graduate, actively practiced law until he reached 65, but confesses he always found special satisfaction in his political and volunteer leadership roles. Virginia, a University of Vermont graduate, worked for several years as a writer, photographer, and editor before their marriage. Busy years of managing the household, raising their children, and being a community volunteer filled the early years of their marriage for her.

In their 50s, John realized he needed a change, so they moved to Burlington to expand this branch office of the law firm he started in St. Johnsbury. That move failed to satisfy him, he says, because "I took a son-of-a-bitch named John Downs with me, and I had to learn to get better acquainted with him." He began to specialize in lobbying, started a novel, and worked with a collaborative group of New England and Russian attorneys. By the time he reached 65 and could afford to retire from his active law practice, he says, "I had a full plate."

After John's retirement, the Downs bought into a Florida mobile home community, expecting to have an active life there during the winter months. They soon had to undo this drastic mistake. Virginia explains, "We were misfits. To us it seemed that people were going around aimlessly with nothing to do but talk by the pool and drink." They decided to live year-round in the small Vermont community where Virginia had roots, but to travel frequently.

John maintains a close relationship with his law firm and is proud of the people he has helped to hire and mentor. Among his many activities, he is a corporate director, a member of the state's Health Policy Council, and writes columns and books. He seems to enjoy the debates that his columns stimulate. John claims he has an "ego condition that likes to be appreciated and keeps him busy." Virginia writes for various organizations and periodicals, usually doing oral histories. Among her many activities, she faithfully participates in the Great Books Program, recently developed a cultural program, and wrote a book related to the town's celebration of its bicentennial. She also belongs to a number of cultural and social groups. Virginia is professional and determinedly independent about her various roles, especially her writing. She is equally committed to being a support and companion to her husband and keeping in close touch with numerous friends. Together, they lead an active social life.

John is analytical about life planning, thinking in terms of five-year plans for his own life. Virginia is probably more intuitive about her decisions. They appear to share equally in their mutual decision-making and encourage each other to pursue his or her own causes and concerns. John looks forward to a scene which emphasizes local activities, additional writing and reading time, and increased opportunities for searching for his spirituality. A reduction in John's and Virginia's activities would hardly result in their being sedentary or reclusive. Both expect to continue their hiking, tennis, and skiing. Virginia seems to feel that she is beginning to achieve a satisfying balance among her family, writing, friendship, and community service roles.

Since neither has real health problems, John finds it hard to think of death. He is concerned about protecting their assets in case Virginia is left alone. She worries about leaving her husband to care for himself, the future of her children, and the possibility of being a burden to them. Recognizing these possibilities, they have put their names on the list for a Continuing Care Retirement Community (CCRC), which they discuss occasionally. Neither believes they would make such a move unless they were unable to manage in their own home or the other died.

By many standards, the Downs have been fortunate. Yet, both speak of frustrations with being unable to help their young adult children lead happy lives and the distance they are from their children and their new grandchild. They compensate by making many positive contributions to people nearby. Some of their relationships have changed because distance, diverging interests, illness or death have separated them from old friends. While there are regrets, John explains that they are drawn to people who "make good use of their older years by doing interesting things, keeping mind and body active, and leading an exciting life." In addition to good health habits and good friends, both Virginia and John emphasize the importance of doing things that really interest them, things that fulfill their individual need for purpose and give each of them a unique identity. As John says, "You have to make your own life."

At first glance, 76-year-old Jack Robertson has the

appearance of a man who has known major losses. He uses a cane because of severe arthritis and has the gaunt look of a man who has lost most of his stomach to cancer and chemotherapy. Yet look again, and you see a lively man whose brown eyes shine with excitement about the work he is doing and who takes great joy in sharing his life with two teenage daughters.

For many years, Jack was an educator, retiring at age 65. By that time, he had been divorced and remarried to a younger woman, from whom he is now divorced, who is the mother of his daughters. Jack made and used films as part of his teaching, but it was only after he retired that he described himself as a documentary filmmaker. He passionately began to pursue his dream of making a series of films entitled "The Quiet Revolution," with the mission of showing others some of "the new discoveries of people throughout the world where people—especially women—are reforming their lives."

For several years, he sought funding to develop and support the team required to do the various technical aspects of the project, which would take the photographers to remote, rural areas of undeveloped and developing countries. He was often rejected, and some of those he originally contacted at various foundations and agencies who had showed interest in his project either retired or moved to other jobs before taking action on his requests for funding. Fortunately, a key person at the Rockefeller Foundation became interested in the "Quiet Revolution" project. Finally, Jack began to get some funding. He launched the ambitious project without knowing how the rest of the money would be raised. Since his first "break," Jack has raised about $2 million for his project and completed six films supported with educational materials.

Some of his films are to be shown in 1994 on public television. The two films I saw, one made in Bangladesh and the other in India, reveal beauty and dignity in the daily lives of very poor people trying to improve their lives. The moving stories are told entirely through visual image, the words of the people, and native music. There is no narration or statement of the theme in either film, although their messages are powerful.

Jack obviously regrets that his health prevented him from doing the actual filming, although he identified all of the settings and stories. He is very grateful for the skillful work of his photographers and editors, who were trained by Jack to know what images he was seeking. In spite of these losses, I came away from our interview and film viewing more aware of gains than losses in the life of this challenged and committed man. Jack Robertson is committed to showing through his films that "the human spirit will triumph through all kinds of adversity." He testifies that in the last 10 years, he has "learned much about the universality of goodness in people, both the rich and the poor." Jack claims it is the support of friends and family that keeps him going during the bad times. Even though his projects and the funding were often difficult to get moving, he says he never felt out of control of his life and work.

Still busy completing the work on the rural films and arranging for their distribution, Jack is already planning a new series. These films will have the same theme, but are to be filmed in urban environments, perhaps in Colombia or Brazil. Then, no doubt, there will be other plans!

Susan and Herb Gallagher are superb examples of aging people who have led far more varied lives than you might guess on first meeting them in their welcoming home or, more likely, in the midst of one of their large gardens. Parents of two sons who live nearby with their growing families, Susan is 78 and Herb is 82. Herb was born on a Vermont farm, where his father died when Herb was 10. Except for a three-year period when a local teacher arranged for Herb to study industrial design at Pratt Institute in Brooklyn, he announces proudly that he has "walked over plowed ground all my life." Herb uses his artistic talent and Pratt training in many practical ways, and several of his beautiful paintings hang in the Gallaghers' living room. For many years, he worked for the U.S. Postal Service, from which he retired at age 65. Herb says he used to be involved in everything—"Boy Scouts, Masons, whatever," but now he doesn't want any part of it. He says, "I guess I was burned out, paid my dues."

Susan grew up on a ranch in Colorado, was sent to college by her parents, and completed graduate work at Columbia before moving to Lyndon State College, where she subsequently met Herb. She says that "I did a lot of different jobs before I retired at age 62. I'd just get comfortable with a job and then I'd be asked to do a different one." These included tasks as varied as starting a laboratory preschool program and serving as acting president of the college. Susan modestly explains, "One thing I could do was not necessarily have all the new ideas, but help people put together their ideas." A former president of many organizations, she says, "I enjoy people and the stimulation of organizations, but I don't need any recognition now. The only real change for me since I was younger is that I am able to be myself. I take who I am and my experiences with me wherever I go." Susan recently retired from the board of the Area Agency for the Aging, but continues to be active on a state advisory board and with retired teachers.

Since retirement, their rural home and garden have become a major focus of the Gallaghers' lives. They often host either family or community groups for meals and fellowship. Both continue to learn about new plants and growing techniques, and they share their produce and flowers freely with others. Herb fears losing his priority activities. He protests, "She says I have to cut out a lot of the things I do, like plant the garden. She doesn't want me to go up on the roof anymore or go out into the woods without telling her where I'm going." He gave up hunting because everybody he used to go with died, but still goes ice fishing. He claims he doesn't go off as far into the woods alone as he used to, admitting "some things I can't do because I am not sure my legs will carry me." Although he may be more reserved than in his earlier days, Herb's well-known wit was evident in his response when I asked him for his priorities before he died. He retorted that he wanted "to be shot by an irate husband."

High priorities for Susan are doing things with their family and "getting all of this stuff around here organized so it won't be a big burden to them, but I don't know if we're going to get that done." Both hope to continue to travel, although not as arduously as in the past. Susan admits the physical losses of aging—not being able to do what you did before and taking longer to do what you can do—are frustrating aspects of aging. She appreciates that "the best thing about aging is you are wiser." Susan believes that you can change and get a new perspective on yourself at any age, with the right kind of counseling and the willingness to open up. Losing one another would most likely be the cause of a major change for Susan or Herb. While Susan and Herb have encouraged the other to follow individual interests, they say their decisions have, for the most part, been mutual. Susan explains: "In order to make decisions or to figure out how to finance something, we've had to talk a lot. We emphasize what we each do well, and our lives have been a cooperative endeavor when we faced a problem." Herb emphasizes that they're not "religious fanatics." Both agree that they try following the major principles in a number of religions, emphasizing concern for others. Susan spoke for Herb as well, saying they've always believed that it was important to decide "the right thing to do."

Ruth Adams was approaching 80 when I interviewed her. Like others with whom I talked, she couldn't figure out why I wanted to talk with her because she doesn't "do anything special." Born in Egypt to Presbyterian missionaries, she attended school there, except for the years when her father was back in the United States between his overseas assignments. Ruth remembers breakfast as the time her father read from the Bible and evenings spent doing handwork while he shared his love of literature, including *The Last Days of Pompeii,* which made her cry. Ruth's work as an occupational therapist in psychiatric hospitals ended because of a chance encounter with a friend studying for his Ph.D. in English. By then past 30, Ruth decided that she, too, wanted to have a job in which she could read and share good literature. The first university department chair she met told her that they were denying her admission to graduate school because as a woman of her age, the best job she could expect to find would be at a "third-rate women's college in Mississippi." Fortunately, the University of Maryland was happy to admit her, she assumes, because they needed teaching assistants. After teaching briefly at two other colleges, Ruth decided she wanted to move to Vermont, where her father served at the East Craftsbury Church before Ruth was of school age.

Following her move, she taught college literature and composition in the state for 13 years before retiring and still spends most of her days and nights as she always has—reading. When we talked, she was eager to discuss a new book by Timothy Ferris on human intelligence. Ruth reports that she knits as she reads and makes most of her own clothes. While she enjoyed her students, she felt no loss in retiring. In fact, she believes that she commands more respect now than she did then. Indeed, it was Ruth who helped me with a usage question as I edited the previous chapters of this book by explaining that a specific word

I was using was "old-fashioned."

Ruth's teaching no longer structures her life, so she is home a good deal. She contentedly lives alone in her farm-style home in a picturesque village, surrounded by familiar objects and stacks of books and periodicals. The upper floor is reserved for sewing and drying her clothes. She confesses to being a great baseball fan, watching every game of the Red Sox on cable television. She is not active in a local church, but occasionally attends community programs and events. When I offered to drive should we be going to the same place in winter weather, her response was, "If it's not safe for me to drive, it's not safe for you either."

In addition to her reading and baseball games, Ruth spends two mornings each week tutoring third graders in writing. Turned down by the first school to which she offered her services for older students, she was welcomed by the principal of a second school. When she first started tutoring children, she wondered how she would deal with nine-year-olds. Now, she says that the methods of teaching writing are just the same with all ages. She asks questions designed to motivate the children to provide supporting details and to organize what they wish to say.

Ruth remains close to her older sister and to her younger brother. She writes to her sister about some of her reading and shares visits with her brother, who lives in England, every year or so. She used to do more traveling, but now finds that making too many transfers or changes tires her. Ruth confesses that she first became aware of herself as aging a few years ago when she realized that she had less stamina for gardening than in previous summers. Her hearing is impaired, although she does not wear a hearing aid, and her eyes have deteriorated. Severe loss of vision would be a difficult change for Ruth to accept. Ruth takes medication for high blood pressure and expects that, since her parents died in their early 60s of heart disease, she, too, will die quietly in her sleep. Death does not seem to worry or preoccupy her. Still, Ruth feels that the "gradual infirmity" of old age is hard to accept. She admits to being "bothered" about the differences in her health, but does not feel "outraged." Ruth observes in her older sister changes that she realizes have also begun in her. While she says she hasn't started to worry about the future, she has started to think about it. Two neighbors check in on her if they fail to see her as usual.

The life of Ruth Adams appears to have had an atypical unity. Although I did not know her in earlier times, the consistency of her priorities and her genteel, but fierce, independence seem to have been the marks of her life since early childhood. Ruth continues to develop and reach out to others, consistently integrating her life around her commitment to literature and family. I cannot imagine that her next life scene will vary much from these motifs.

Clark Taylor, 85, remains remarkably active, interested, and caring throughout his Third Act. Clark lives in his own apartment in a new CCRC on Cape Cod, where he became one of the first residents within a few years after the death of his wife, Myrtle. Married for 55 years, they had planned to make this move together. He admitted that he spent several months after his wife's death checking with other men who had lost their "mates" to see how they coped. He also shared cooking meals with some for awhile. While enjoying the companionship, he was not satisfied with this arrangement. Clark also considered and rejected staying in his Cape Cod house and getting help or finding someone with whom to live.

Since childhood, Clark has been part of a family tradition of commitment to the Christian church as a community of persons who share and support each other. He now seems to regard his relationships and activities with others in his CCRC as taking place within such a community. His other major relationships are with his three children and their families, an accomplished and politically diverse group who sometimes challenge his flexibility. He and Myrtle traveled considerably following his retirement, often organizing their trips around their children's locations. Since two of his children and their families now live relatively close by, he need not travel far to see them, although he still occasionally visits relatives across the country.

Clark says that he feels healthier at 85 than before he retired at age 60 from management at Illinois Bell Telephone. After completing a bachelor's degree in night school during the Depression years, he spent his middle adult years riding trains into his Chicago office from their suburban home combined with numerous church and community leadership roles. Both his developing glaucoma and a long siege of company strikes made early retirement attractive. The financial loss he took to retire early has never caused him to regret the decision.

Clark considers himself a "doer," not an "in-depth thinker." As the first president of the community's resident board, Clark provided leadership in deciding how to structure group life in their new community, obviously sensing the significance of establishing policies that would serve everyone over time. His activities in developing this new community cover everything from gardening to governance. He participates in numerous community events, as well as his daily walks, swimming class, and a group exercise class. Another project has been to photograph new residents and special programs. When asked why he does all of this, he says it just "seemed like we ought to be doing something. Some residents have a tendency to stay in their apartments. We try to get them to come out."

You hear little about loss from Clark Taylor, except a consistent awareness of the absence of the mate with whom he would like to have shared recent years. Clark has made close women friends in the community with whom he often shares meals, a hug, or a backrub; however, he says he has never wanted to marry again. He does not fear death, but is adamant about staying out of the nursing home section. This motivates his exercise and dietary control, and he proudly reports blood pressure and cholesterol counts younger men would envy. Placement in the nursing home represents loss of independence to Clark. He is glad to be able to continue driving, although he recently promised his children that he would not drive at night or any farther than Cape Cod.

Clark sees himself as much more relaxed about things than he used to be; yet, he still believes in the importance of "patterns." He described his need to find a new pattern for both daily living and social relations after his wife's death. And, he follows a "regular pattern" of rising and doing his daily chores, as well as exercising. Both his mind and his body stay active. In fact, Clark telephoned me after our interview to point out that we had not discussed his interests in national and world affairs. He tries to read a balanced selection of daily and weekly periodicals as well as to watch television news. The key themes for the aging years of this friendly, gracious gentleman appear to be: stay physically and mentally active, be orderly, look ahead, and be alert to the needs of others.

As I worked on this book, I met many professionals whose daily jobs are to care for and share with the elderly. The elderly men or women are apt to be nearing their own deaths, experiencing severe personal illness, or facing the approaching death of a spouse. Their admirable ways of dealing with life—and death—in their closing scenes are worth noting. Many women, especially those in their eighth or ninth decades, live alone and depend on a team of persons to assist them to stay in their own homes.

Rita LaFerriere, a nurse who provides rural residents

with a variety of medical and educational services, recently completed a study of wellness in rural women past age 85. She shared some of her findings with me, as well as these summary comments from one woman she interviewed on several occasions:

"I'm just ordinary people—there's nothing special about me! I've lived for 92 years, all but a couple of them right here in this town. Lots of things have changed over those years. I've seen family farms disappear, electricity and airplanes introduced, and have known personal losses.

"I've been a widow for many years. When your husband dies it takes half of your life. You have to look out for yourself, and you've got to keep going. It's quite an adjustment to live just for yourself.

"I've experienced my share of health problems even though my health is pretty good for someone my age. Once I had a ruptured appendix and was in the hospital for almost a year. I've broken my hip, my arm, my shoulder, my pelvis, and had a couple of heart attacks and a slight stroke. I've even been in a nursing home for awhile twice, but I've always been able to come home because of my family's willingness to help one another. I think older people tend to think about their illnesses, their ailments, and I try not to. I try to look on the bright side of things. I do counted cross-stitch, make small items for church sales, talk to friends, or bake bread. These kinds of work are good for you.

"Staying active and eating right are important, too. Having good food and not always going to the store to buy it matters. Determination to do for yourself and not being waited on help to keep you independent. One of the hardest things I had to give up was my driver's license. I stopped driving when I was 86. Then I had to ask somebody to drive me, but before I always liked to just step out and go somewhere, just where I wanted to go and not be dependent on someone to take me. I miss that."

Herbert Perry, himself thinking of retiring for the second time at age 65, recalls how impressed he was early in his ministry when he called in one home. There he met a man whom he came to regard highly, and whose funeral he would later prepare. According to Herb, the old man was nearly blind, and his wife was dying of a painful disease in an upper room of the home. When the young pastor tried to say something about the circumstances that were closing in on them, the aged man just brushed all that aside. Instead, as they stood at the door, he said, "We ought to be profoundly grateful for having been allowed to live at so great a time as this." Herb points out that in spite of his blindness and with pain all about him, and with sorrow awaiting him, that man's "basic disposition of grace and gratitude still prevailed."

These Third Act people are immeasurably more complex than we can know through these quick glimpses. Each is unique, but there are astounding similarities in their emphases on keeping active, caring about someone or something, and staying in control of their own lives. When asked how they managed to be resilient when facing changes, few could tell me more than that they'd always had to face problems or "do for themselves." As we discussed how people decide to make changes, the couples agreed that they talked things through and made mutual, rather than one-sided, decisions. While often proud of their past achievements and holding prized memories of times and relationships during their first two acts, these people focus on the present and the immediate future in their Third Act scenes. More than once I was asked, "What are you going to do next after you finish this book?" These women and men emphasize living each new day fully—warmly meeting new people, sharing freely what they know and do, and applying current information to keeping themselves as healthy as possible.

These are strong, independent individuals; however, they seem to have developed some type of support system of family, neighbors, friends, and professionals on whom they can call if they should need help. Some belong to religious groups, but even those people are much more committed to caring, stimulating relations with others than to a religion or institution. No one seems to fear dying, although many are quite concerned about their possibilities for becoming incapable of managing daily tasks—and thus, dependent on others.

KEY THEMES AND PRINCIPLES FOR LIFE'S THIRD ACT

Joseph Joubert once said, "I had to grow old to learn what I wanted to know, and I should need to be young to say well what I know." I agree with the first part of his comment and hope that the second part does not apply to me. If I had thought I could adequately tell you in a few pages about all of the themes and principles for taking control of your Third Act, I would not have written the first six chapters! I used the stories because it is all too easy to ignore the realities of typical challenges to women and men over 50 if we separate them from the daily lives of people. I believe that we often understand ourselves better and deal with our own life situations more effectively by having examples. You probably saw yourself or someone you love in one or more of the characters you met in this book. Some of their experiences may have seemed uncomfortably familiar to you. Their relative successes or failures in managing transitions may have inspired you to stay in control as you face change in your own life. Here is a concise version of the main ideas.

Believing That You Can Grow And Be In Control Makes It Possible

Some people stay productive and joyful for all or most of their lives, while others seem to withdraw from society or become uninterested and inactive. People who believe they can develop and change during their mature years generally do so, while persons who think they cannot change in the face of new circumstances after they are 50, or any other age, do not grow and adapt. They just suffer, and often make life unpleasant for the rest of us as well.

Older people typically are not physically or mentally incompetent. Most of us are not even unpleasant! Some men and women do live many years with severe chronic conditions, such as heart disease, cancer, diabetes, or loss of limb. Most experience only a few months or years of chronic illness. We generally have the capacity to remain in control throughout these periods, if we have sufficient determination and understanding about ourselves as we age, and have arranged for others to manage affairs when we can't. Research indicates that feeling in control of your life can improve both physical and mental well-being.

Knowing Both What To Expect And How To Handle Changes Makes Aging Easier

Change is a constant in our world rather than a crisis to be avoided. We tend to be optimistic about the changes we face as children and young adults, and usually, even those which occur in mid-life. Nevertheless, we're often frustrated and fearful about handling the changes we expect to occur after age 50. Yet, when you know the realities of aging and use sensible guidelines for living those years with control and dignity, you have an excellent chance of handling changes well and continuing to live happily.

We do not require prophets or crystal balls to tell us that

either we or those close to us will have significant economic, physical, or emotional losses. That is the stuff of life. Yes, the losses most of us experience as we age are often permanent and, therefore, especially difficult to accept. As John Burroughs said years ago, "Time does not become sacred to us until we have lived it, until it has passed over us and taken with it a part of ourselves." Still, the inevitable losses of our mature years normally can be balanced until the end of life by new opportunities and insights if we grasp those new opportunities and respond according to our fresh insights.

Certain Experiences And Concerns Are Common To Particular Age Ranges

Almost all men and women know disappointments and losses well before age 50, since from childhood we have given up certain roles and relationships in order to take on others as we matured. While we are not genetically programmed to have specific physical, financial, or social changes take place at precise ages, people face remarkably similar challenges over the years. Many significant changes are age-related—retirement, children leaving home, changes in vision or hearing, and the death or illness of parents, partners, and close friends. We may confront retirement, our children reaching adulthood, death of our parents, divorce or our spouse's death, and moves from one community to another—all before we reach age 60.

Occasionally we forget that contrasted with these losses are the considerable freedoms and new opportunities which are either presented to us or which we can help to create during these years. Finally, we can stop climbing job ladders and be relieved from the daily responsibilities of parenting. Many of us have sufficient economic stability and health to begin new work, learn new things, develop new relationships, and especially, to play—a luxury our structured young adult and middle years often did not permit.

Life For Each Of Us Is Comparable To Playing A Role In A Stage Production

For many people, life has at least three major sections, like acts in a play. Childhood and the student years represent the First Act, a formative and dependent period. For some, the first act ends around age 20, although others are closer to 30 before becoming fully adult in the view of society. Economic independence and regular parental and community responsibilities typically dominate our roles in the Second Act. During this period, we must earn, save, and supervise, often delaying personal goals. Retirement from full-time employment and regular parental and community tasks usually initiates the Third Act. While more and more people live until their mid-80s or later, the Third Act begins for an increasing number in their early 50s, because they have fewer children and retire younger than in earlier decades.

Many mature adults move into their Third Act, initiating and implementing plans for new life scenes, with notable grace. By contrast, some women and men either deny they've reached these scenes in their life dramas or exhibit an ungraceful reluctance to assume new roles, often blaming their employers, spouses, or others for their situations.

Living Well In The Third Act Requires A Series Of Roles And Scripts—Not Just One Plan

Most of us understand that we must plan how to pay for our years after retirement from full-time employment and that deciding where to live is a critical step. But, beyond that, many fail to plan—and some are devastated when their general plans don't seem to be working. Because change is constant, planning as we age must also be a continuing, conscious process, not a one-time event.

Periodically, we must—either by choice or unforseen circumstances—move into new scenes. Whenever those changes occur, we have to develop new life scripts. Even when there are no major changes, effective living calls for regular reviews of our situations as well as occasional crisis revisions, just as any well-run organization requires.

Good planning will not, of course, produce the same script for each of us. Forbid that all 58-year-old women decided to run for political office or open antique stores! Or that every retired man began baking bread or producing wooden toys! Our chosen scripts and roles must consider our personalities and situations and also the needs and preferences of those close to us. In addition, the possibilities for our next scripts depend on the options still available at the end of our previous scenes.

Good plans for the scenes ahead will be realistic ones, not fantasy. Our scripts must be based on a real understanding of our unique challenges and opportunities at the time, or we will not be very successful in playing our roles. While our plans need to include others who share our daily lives, each person has to create and act his or her own script. Maintaining a separate identity is extremely important to staying in control at all ages.

Good Planning Requires Accurate Information And Effective Planning Strategies

You already know and use several common strategies for dealing with transitions and can easily learn those you have not yet tried. Professional advisors are helpful and should be used according to your needs for expert information, skills, or objectivity. Still, only you can assume personal responsibility for recognizing that change is occurring either in you or in your environment and, then, for managing your transitions.

The eight strategies for taking control during your transitions, which are presented in chapter 6, are classified as:

1. Reaching out to others;
2. Reconsidering your situation;
3. Opening yourself to the possibility of changing;
4. Ending some of your current activities
   and emphases;
5. Searching for your new purpose and challenges;
6. Deciding which role to take on next;
7. Planning the action for your new scene; and
8. Beginning the scene.

Don't Become A Slave To Your Planning!

By the time we reach our Third Acts, most of us realize that life is too short and too precious to be spent in worrying about everything we do, making detailed lists of tasks, and blaming ourselves for all that seems to go wrong. Please do not think that is what I am advocating here. It's not that complicated. My even shorter summary of basic ideas for taking control of your mature years follows:

- Take pleasure and pride in what you have already accomplished;
- Consider your challenges as ways to continue growing and changing;
- "Make change your friend, not your enemy."
  —President Clinton;
- Draw on your own experience and the examples and ideas in this book as you face future changes;
- Get yourself out of a scene you do not like or cannot play well;
- Try to spend most of each day doing what you highly value;
- Stay as mentally and physically active as you possibly can;

- Be the kind of caring and interested friend you want to have;
- Be assertive and clear when important needs are not being met; and
- Accept the concerns and assistance of others without losing your own sense of value and control.

We each have continuing personal struggles to maintain control over our lives. Sometimes we lack the strength or courage to make the changes that offer us possibilities for greater pleasure and peace. It is my fervent hope that this book has encouraged you to undertake new roles and scenes in your life. As Phillip Vernier, a French pastor, once advised, "Do not wait for great strength before setting out, for immobility will weaken you further. Do not wait to see very clearly before starting: one has to walk toward the light. Have you strength enough to take this first step? Courage enough to accomplish this little tiny act...the necessity of which is apparent to you? Take this step! Perform this act! You will be astonished to feel that the effort accomplished, instead of having exhausted your strength, has doubled it—and that you already see more clearly what you have to do next."

Resources

In addition to books and articles, numerous government and private organizations offer information and services to help you plan your mature years. Many of the national organizations listed here also have state or regional agencies that they may refer you to for specific assistance. Similarly, every state has an *Office on Aging,* which will direct you to local agencies that serve as resources for the aging.

One excellent place to start your research is your regional *Area Agency on Aging.* Also, local telephone books usually provide a "Guide to Services" that includes crisis contacts as well as various categories of services helpful to those making life changes; some even list an "Aging Information and Referral" toll-free number.

Many of the organizations, associations, and agencies featured on the following pages exist expressly to assist the growing numbers of mature persons in the United States. Use them! Please note these listings are provided for informational purposes only and no endorsement is intended by either the author or publisher of this book. Since organizations sometimes move, it's a good idea to call and confirm an address before sending a letter or making a visit.

This resource guide is designed to help you start your search by pointing you in the right direction. Thus, the following list is organized by broad categories of interest and need—and is in no way intended to represent a comprehensive catalog of every available resource.

BEGINNING NEW ACTIVITIES: VOLUNTEERING, WORK, AND TRAVEL

Becoming A Volunteer

Habitat for Humanity International
21 Habitat Street
Americus, GA 31709

International Executive Service Corps
8 Stamford Forum
Stamford, CT 06901

Service Corps of Retired Executives
Small Business Administration
1441 L Street, NW
Washington, DC 20416

Other sources to consider:
Information about Senior Community Service Employment may be available from your Area Agency on Aging; also, look for the Retired Senior Volunteer Program (RSVP) listing in your local telephone directory.

To share recreation, companionship, and meals with others over 60, contact your Area Agency on Aging and ask about senior centers and meal sites.

To be a foster grandparent or senior companion, contact:
ACTION Older American Volunteer Programs
1100 Vermont Avenue, NW
6th Floor
Washington, DC 20525
(202) 606-5135

Finding New Jobs

Center for Entrepreneurial Management
311 Main Street
Worcester, MA 01608

Project 55
20 Nassau Street
Princeton, NJ 08542

Senior Career Planning and Placement Service
(Executive Placement)
257 Park Avenue South
New York, NY 10010
(212) 529-6660

Other sources to consider:
Operation ABLE for Older Job Seekers exists in the states of
Arkansas, California, Massachusetts, Michigan, Nebraska,
New York, and Vermont. Contact:
Dorothy Miaso
36 South Wabash Street #1133
Chicago, IL 60603

Also, Forty Plus Clubs offer job searching assistance to
those over age 40. See job listings in your local newspaper.

Starting Your Own Business

Center for Home-Based Businesses
Truman College
1145 West Wilson
Chicago, IL 60640
(312) 989-6112

Elder Craftsmen
135 East 65th Street
New York, NY 10021
(212) 861-5260

Other sources to consider:
A *Franchise Opportunities Handbook* is available at your
area government printing office bookstore or from the U.S.
Government Printing Office. Call (202) 783-3238 for current
price and to order.

Traveling When You're Older

Many organizations offer travel services designed especially for older persons. Here are some of the better known:
AARP Land and Air Tours
(800) 927-0111

AARP Cruises
(800) 745-4567

Grand Circle Travel
347 Congress Street
Boston, MA 02210
(800) 221-2610

SCI National Retirees of America
134 Franklin Street
Hempstead, NY 11550
(800) 645-3382

Grand Travel (Intergenerational Vacations)
6900 Wisconsin Avenue, #706
Chevy Chase, MD 20815
(800) 247-7651

Walking the World (Outdoor Adventures)
P.O. Box 1186
Fort Collins, CO 80522
(303) 224-0449

Other sources and travel tips:
To get on the mailing list for Elderhostel, which conducts educational programs throughout the U.S. and the world for persons over 60, contact:
Elderhostel
75 Federal Street
Boston, MA 02110

Before preparing to travel in the U.S., get maps and detailed information about what to see and do. Write to the offices of tourism in each state you wish to visit.

Free admission to federal parks, monuments, and recreation areas is available with a "Golden Age Passport," offered by most federally operated recreation facilities. You must show proof that you are at least 62 years old and either a citizen or permanent resident of the U.S.

Traveling abroad typically requires passports, visas, and vaccinations. For passports, contact your U.S. Post Office or call (202) 647-0518 at least six months before departure.

If you're not sure whether you'll need a visa, contact:
U.S. Department of State
Citizens Emergency Center
2201 C Street, NW, #4811
Washington, DC 20520
(202) 647-5225
(Request the brochure *Travel Tips for Senior Citizens.*)

To find out what vaccinations you need, contact your local Department of Health.

BECOMING AN ACTIVE CITIZEN

Stay in touch by mail or phone with your elected representatives, and vote in each election. Addresses and telephone numbers are available from your local telephone book, the League of Women Voters, or state legislative clerk. Consider joining:

Concerned Seniors for Better Government
815 16th Street, NW
6th Floor
Washington, DC 20036

To stay informed and improve conditions for older persons, join one or more of the national, state, or local groups that represent senior citizens. (See also the "Planning in General" section.)

MANAGING YOUR MONEY AND INSURANCE

To reach the Veterans Administration Regional Offices, or to inquire about benefits and insurance, call (800) 669-8477; hearing-impaired person using a TDD, call (800) 829-4833.

To contact the Social Security's Nationwide Toll-Free Service, call (800) 772-1213.

For guides on nursing homes, home care, and health financing, contact:

The United Seniors Health Cooperative
1331 H Street, NW, #500
Washington, DC 20005

To receive a long-term care insurance guide, contact:

AARP Fulfillment
601 E Street, NW
Washington, DC 20049

Information on filing for Medicare is available at Medicare State Claim Offices. Check your telephone book for the toll-free number.

For help with selecting insurance policies and protection of your rights as a policyholder, contact State Insurance Regulators.

For information on reverse mortgages, contact:
American Association of Retired Persons
Home Equity Conversion Center
1909 K Street, NW
Washington, DC 20049
(202) 728-4355

For information on sale leaseback arrangements:
National Center for Home Equity Conversion
110 East Main Street, #605
Madison, WI 53703

To get help with tax questions, or volunteer your own expertise, contact:
Tax-Aide Program
AARP Program Department
601 E Street, NW
Washington, DC 20049
(202) 434-2277

For information on tax differences among states, contact AARP and ask for the *Relocation Tax Guide: State Tax Information for Relocation Decisions.*

To obtain federal tax forms and publications, call (800) 829-3676; for assistance on tax law and tax preparation, call IRS Telephone Assistance Service, (800) 829-1040.

Older persons often can receive discounts on a wide variety of goods and services. Ask transportation, phone and utility companies, movie theaters, restaurants, museums, banks, colleges, and recreational facilities if they offer a Senior Citizen discount and watch for "specials."

MANAGING YOUR HEALTH

Starting or Expanding Your Exercise Program

National Association for Human Development
1424 16th Street, NW
Washington, DC 20036
(202) 328-2191

National Senior Sports Association
10560 Main Street, #205
Fairfax, VA 22030
(703) 385-7540

President's Council on Physical Fitness and Sports
450 Fifth Street, NW, #7103
Washington, DC 20001
(202) 272-3430

Coping with Common Health Concerns

The following addresses and phone numbers will put you in touch with experts familiar with the more common health concerns of older adults.
Health Information Center
Office of Disease Prevention and Health Promotion
P.O. Box 1133
Washington, DC
(301) 565-4167 or (800) 336-4797

National Institute on Aging Information Center
P.O. Box 8057
Gaithersburg, MD 20857
(301) 495-3455

American Cancer Society
1599 Clifton Road, NE
Atlanta, GA 30329
(800) 227-2345

American Heart Association
7320 Greenville Avenue
Dallas, TX 75231
(214) 750-5397

American Diabetes Association
1660 Duke Street
Alexandria, VA 22314
(800) 232-34723

Arthritis Foundation
P.O. Box 1900
Atlanta, GA 30327
(800) 283-7800

National Chronic Pain Outreach Association
7979 Old Georgetown Road, #100
Bethesda, MD 20814
(301) 652-4948

Alcoholism and Drug Addiction Treatment Center
(800) 382-4357

Alcoholics Anonymous
P.O. Box 459, Grand Central Station
New York, NY 10163
(212) 686-1100

Cocaine Abuse Hotline
(800) 262-2463

National Women's Health Network
1325 G Street, NW
Washington, DC 20005
(202) 347-1140
(Also check for women's wellness centers in
your community.)

Alzheimer's Disease and Related Disorders Association
70 East Lake Street, # 600
Chicago, IL 60601
(800) 272-3900
[In Illinois, call (800) 527-6037]

USDA's Meat and Poultry Hotline
(800) 535-4555
[In District of Columbia, call (202) 447-3333]

Hearing Helpline
(800) 327-9355
[In Virginia, call (703) 642-0580]

National Institute of Mental Health
Public Inquiries Branch
Parklawn Building, Room 15C-05
5600 Fishers Lane
Rockville, MD 20857
(301) 443-4513

American Association for Geriatric Psychiatry
P.O. Box 376-A
Greenbelt, MD 20770
(301) 220-0952

American Psychological Association
1200 17th Street, NW
Washington, DC 20036
(202) 955-7600

American Dental Association
211 East Chicago Avenue
Chicago, IL 60611
(312) 440-2860

Foundation for Glaucoma Research
490 Post Street, #830
San Francisco, CA 94102
(415) 986-3162

Other sources to check:
For advice on selecting and purchasing medical supplies
and equipment, contact your local hospital or medical
center, the Area Agency on Aging, or the Better Business
Bureau, rather than relying on the phone book or having a
salesperson call on you.

To identify your state's home care association, contact:
National Association for Home Care
519 C Street, NE
Stanton Park
Washington, DC 20002
(202) 547-7424

For a comprehensive geriatric assessment, contact your
family physician, your local Area Agency on Aging, your
local hospital's internal medicine department, or a nearby
veterans hospital.

For hospice information and local referrals:
Hospice Association of America
519 C Street, NE
Washington, DC 20002
(202) 547-5263

National Hospice Organization
1901 N. Fort Myer Drive, #902
Arlington, VA 22209
(703) 243-5900

SELECTING HOUSING

General information on housing options is available in a free housing packet provided by:
AARP HO7 Program Department Correspondence Unit
1909 K Street, NW
Washington, DC 20049

For information on retirement communities, contact:
American Association of Homes for the Aging
901 E Street, NW, #500
Washington, DC 20004
(202) 508-9442

A checklist to aid you in evaluating assisted living facilities is available from:
Assisted Living Facility Association of America
9401 Lee Highway, #402
Fairfax, CA 94930

For information on senior apartments, contact your local housing authority or regional housing and urban development office.

For advice on adult day care programs, contact your Area Agency on Aging.

Information on selecting a nursing home is available from:
American Health Care Association
1201 L Street, NW
Washington, DC 20005
(202) 842-4444

Other sources to consider:
Customized guidance in selecting retirement living options
is provided by:
The Transitions Group, Inc.
P.O. Box 239
East Burke, VT 05832
(802) 626-8321

National Shared Housing Resource Center
431 Pine Street
Burlington, VT 05401
(802) 862-2727

HANDLING CONTRACTS AND LEGAL ARRANGEMENTS

For information about Durable Power of Attorney and
lawyers in your area, contact:
National Academy of Elder Law Attorneys
655 N. Alvernon Way, #108
Tucson, AZ 85711
(602) 881-4005

For information about legal rights:
National Senior Citizens Law Center
1815 H Street, NW, #700
Washington, DC 20006
(202) 887-5280

For a written guide to legal matters of aging, write to:
AARP, Legal Counsel for the Elderly
P.O. Box 96474
Washington, DC 20090

Other sources to consider:
Free or low-cost legal services are available from Legal Aid and other legal services offices; check your local telephone book or your Area Agency on Aging.

Records of births, marriages, divorces, or deaths can be found through your state's Department of Health or vital records office (for New York City records, contact the city's Department of Health).

Help for an abused older person is available through your state's Adult Protective Services or your local police department. Check your telephone directory or call the 911 emergency number.

For instructions on filing a complaint of age or sex discrimination, call the Equal Employment Opportunity Commission, (800) 669-4000.

To file a complaint about a local business, contact your local or state consumer protection office. Concerns about fraud or misrepresentation by a national company should be addressed to:
National Consumers League
815 Fifteenth Street, NW, #928
Washington, DC 20005
(202) 639-8140

To report mail fraud or ask about mail-order sales:
 Chief Postal Inspector
 P.O. Box 96096
 Washington, DC 20006-6096
 (202) 636-2300

To donate your body for transplantation or research,
you may register with:
 The Living Bank
 P.O. Box 6725
 Houston, TX 77265
 (800) 528-2971

For information and sample copies of Living Wills, contact:
 Society for the Right to Die
 250 West 57th Street
 New York, NY 10107
 (212) 246-6962

Sample healthcare documents, and instructions for their
completion, are available from
 Choice in Dying
 200 Varick Street
 New York, NY 10014
 (212) 366-5540

Information on Preplanning Funerals

 Continental Association of Funeral and Memorial
 Societies, Inc.
 6900 Lost Lake Road
 Egg Harbor, WI 54209
 (800) 458-5563

 Association of Funeral and Memorial Societies
 20001 S Street
 Washington, DC 20009
 (202) 745-0634

GROWING PERSONALLY

Opportunities for Creative Aging

Assistance for Recently Widowed Women
Displaced Homemaker Network
1411 K Street, NW, #930
Washington, DC 20005
(202) 628-6767

Beverly Foundation
70 South Lake Avenue, #750
Pasadena, CA 91101
(818) 792-2292

Continuing Your Education

For college courses at reduced or no tuition, contact your area college, or:
The Institute of Lifetime Learning, AARP
1909 K Street, NW
Washington, DC 20049

To learn and communicate by using a computer:
SeniorNet
University of San Francisco
San Francisco, CA 94117
(415) 666-6505

To find out about books, magazines, video and audio tapes, and often artwork on loan—as well as participate in special activities—go to your local library.

To learn while traveling, see Elderhostel listing under "Traveling When You're Older," page 172.

Other sources and ideas to consider:
To meet new people and work for causes you care about, become active in organizations for retired persons that represent your former career field(s).

To share your experience with children and young people, volunteer to tutor in schools or share a talent through a religious or community program for youth.

To share the traditions and principles of your ethnic, racial, or religious group, find a local association that fosters pride in your group, or contact a national organization that represents your heritage, and ask for information on area programs.

To pursue intellectual or personal interests, join a group— or start your own—of people interested in exploring similar issues. Such groups offer the opportunity to share your leadership skills and get ideas from the group for readings, films, or tapes that will foster group discussions.

To seek answers to questions of meaning and spirituality, use articles and books by such twentieth century authors as Ernest Becker, Frederick Buechner, Henri Nouen, Sam Keen, Victor Frankl, M. Scott Peck, Paul Tillich, Eric Fromm, and Harold Kushner, as well as fiction and classical literature.

PLANNING IN GENERAL

To locate federal agencies that address specific needs and services, contact:
Federal Information Center
P.O. Box 600
Cumberland, MD 21502-0600
Phone numbers vary by time zone:
Alaska (800) 729-8003

Mountain Time (800) 359-3997
Eastern Standard Time (800) 347-1997
Pacific Time (800) 726-4995
Central Time (800) 366-2998

Administration on Aging
Department of Health and Human Services
330 Independence Avenue, SW
Washington, DC 20201
(202) 619-0724

Membership Organizations for Seniors

American Association of Retired Persons
601 E Street, NW
Washington, DC 20049
(202) 434-2277

Gray Panthers
1424 Sixteenth Street, NW, #602
Washington, DC 20036
(202) 387-3111

National Alliance for Senior Citizens, Inc.
1700 Eighteenth Street, NW, #401
Washington, DC 20009
(202) 968-0017

National Association for the Hispanic Elderly
3325 Wilshire Boulevard, #800
Los Angeles, CA 90010
(213) 487-1922

National Association of Retired Federal Employees
1533 Hampshire Avenue, NW
Washington, DC 20036
(202) 234-0832

National Caucus and Center on Black Aged, Inc.
1424 K Street, NW, #500
Washington, DC 20005
(202) 637-8400

National Committee to Preserve
Social Security and Medicare
2000 K Street, NW #800
Washington, DC 20006
(202) 822-9459

National Council on Aging
409 Third Street, SW
Washington, DC 20024
(202) 479-1200

National Indian Council on Aging, Inc.
6400 Uptown Boulevard, NE, #510W
Albuquerque, NM 87110
(505) 888-3302

Older Women's League
730 Eleventh Street, NW, #300
Washington, DC 20001
(202) 783-6686

PLANNING FOR SPECIAL NEEDS

Care Managers in Your Area

National Association of Professional Geriatric
Care Managers
655 North Alvernon Way, #108
Tucson, AZ 85711
(602) 881-8008

Home Care Agencies and Hospices

National Association for Home Care
519 C Street, NE
Stanton Park
Washington, DC 20002
(202) 547-7424

National Home Caring Council
235 Park Avenue South
New York, NY 10003
(212) 674-4990

Services for the Blind

American Council for the Blind, Inc.
15 West 16th Street
New York, NY 10011
(800) 424-8666

Help for Deaf Persons

National Information Center on Deafness
Gallaudet University
800 Florida Avenue, NE
Washington, DC 20002
(202) 651-5051 (TDD—5052)

To contact U.S. government offices, call:
Federal Government TDD Assistance
(800) 855-1155

Assistance for Older Persons with Disabilities

National Rehabilitation Information Center
8455 Colesville Road, #935
Silver Spring, MD 20910
(800) 346-2742

To inquire about dogs for persons with disabilities other than blindness:
Canine Companions for Independence
P.O. Box 446
Santa Rosa, CA 95402
(707) 528-0830

To learn more about services for persons with disabilities, contact state vocational and rehabilitation agencies; also check under "vocational" or "rehabilitation" listings in the government section of your local phone book.

References

GENERAL

Bridges, William. *Transitions: Making Sense of Life's Changes.* Reading, MA: Addison-Wesley Publishing Company, 1980.

Chopra, Deepak. *Ageless Body, Timeless Mind: The Quantum Alternative to Growing Old.* New York: Harmony Books, 1993.

Friedan, Betty. *The Fountain of Age.* New York: Simon & Schuster, 1993.

Gerzon, Mark. *Coming Into Our Own: The Adult Metamorphis.* New York: Delacorte Publishers, 1991.

Kotre, John and Elizabeth Hall. *Seasons of Life: Our Dramatic Journey From Birth To Death.* Boston: Little, Brown and Company, 1990.

Leshan, Eda. *It's Better to Be Over the Hill Than Under It: Thoughts on Life Over Sixty.* New York: Newmarket Press, 1990.

Rubin, Lillian. *Women of a Certain Age: The Midlife Search for Self.* New York: Harper & Row, 1979.

Scarf, Maggie. *Unfinished Business: Pressure Points in the Lives of Women.* New York: Doubleday & Company, Inc., 1980.

Sheehy, Gail. *Pathfinders.* New York: William Morrow and Company, Inc., 1981.

Siegal, Bernie S. *Peace, Love and Healing.* New York: Harper & Row, 1989.

Steinem, Gloria. *Revolution From Within: A Book of Self-Esteem.* Boston: Little, Brown and Company, 1992.

Viorst, Judith. *Necessary Losses.* New York: Ballantine Books, 1987.

HOW TO

Anderson-Ellis, Eugenia. *Aging Parents and You.* New York: MasterMedia Limited, 1988.

Ballard, Jack and Phoebe Ballard. *Beating the Age Game: Redefining Retirement.* New York: MasterMedia Limited, 1993.

Barrowclough, Christine and Ian Fleming. *Goal Planning with Elderly People.* Manchester, UK: Manchester University Press, 1986.

Brown, David. *The Rest of Your Life is The Best of Your Life.* New York: Barricade Books Inc., 1993.

Gross, Andrea. *Shifting Gears: Planning a New Strategy for Midlife.* New York: Crown Publishers, Inc., 1991.

Petras, Kathryn and Ross Petras. *The Only Retirement Guide You'll Ever Need.* New York: Poseidon Press, 1991.

Silverstone, Barbara and Helen Kandel Hyman. *You and Your Aging Parent.* New York: Pantheon Books, 1976.

Skala, Ken. *American Guidance for Seniors.* Fourth ed., Falls Church, VA: American Guidance, Inc., 1992.

Teal, Janice and Phyllis Schneider. *Straight Talk on Women's Health: How to Get the Health Care You Deserve!* New York: MasterMedia Limited, 1993.

Tilson, David, ed. *Aging in Place: Supporting the Frail Elderly in Residential Environments.* Professional Books on Aging. Glenview, IL: Scott, Foresman and Company, 1990.

Vicker, Ray. *The Dow Jones-Irwin Guide to Retirement Planning.* Second ed., Homewood, IL: Dow Jones-Irwin, 1987.

POLICY AND RESEARCH

Abel, Emily K. *Who Cares for the Elderly? Public Policy and the Experiences of Adult Daughters.* Philadelphia: Temple University Press, 1991.

Allen, Jessie and Allan Pifer, ed. *Women on the Front Lines: Meeting the Challenge of an Aging America.* Southport, CT: Urban Press Institute, 1993.

Butler, Robert N. *Why Survive? Being Old in America.* New York: Harper & Row, 1975.

Butler, Robert N. and Herbert P. Gleason. *Productive Aging.* New York: Springer-Verlag, 1985.

Callahan, Daniel. *Setting Limits: Medical Goals in an Aging Society.* New York: Simon and Schuster, 1987.

Cockerham, William C. *This Aging Society.* Englewood Cliffs, NJ: Prentice Hall, 1991.

Esposito, Joseph L. *The Obsolete Self: Philosophical Dimensions of Aging.* Berkeley: University of California Press, 1987.

Gould, Roger. *Transformation: Growth and Change in Adult Life.* New York: Simon & Schuster, 1978.

Halpern, Ron. *Quiet Desperation: The Truth About Successful Men.* New York: Warner Books, 1988.

Harrison, Allen F. and Robert M. Bramson. *Styles of Thinking.* Garden City, NY: Anchor Press/Doubleday, 1982.

Heilbrun, Carolyn G. *Writing a Woman's Life.* New York: W.W. Norton, 1988.

Hill, Percy H. *Making Decisions: A Multidisciplinary Introduction.* Advanced Book Program, Reading, MA: Addison-Wesley Publishing Company, 1979.

Hudson, Frederic M. *The Adult Years: Mastering the Art of Self-Renewal.* San Francisco: Jossey-Bass, 1991.

Kalish, Richard A. *Late Adulthood: Perspectives on Human Development.* Monterey, CA: Brooks/Cole Publishing Company, 1975.

Kaufman, Sharon R. *The Ageless Self: Sources of Meaning in Late Life.* Madison, WI: University of Wisconsin Press, 1986.

Laslett, Peter. *A Fresh Map of Life: The Emergence of the Third Age.* London: Wiedenfield and Nicholson, 1989.

Levinson, Daniel and others. *The Seasons of a Man's Life.* New York: Alfred A. Knopf, 1978.

Lowenthal, Margery and others. *Four Stages of Life.* San Francisco: Jossey-Bass, 1975.

Lowenthal, Marjorie Fiske and David A. Chiriboga. *Change and Continuity in Adult Life.* San Francisco: Jossey-Bass Publishers, 1990.

Ory, Marcia G. and Ronald P. Abeles. *Aging, Health, and Behavior.* Newbury Park, CA: Sage Publishers, 1992.

Palmore, Erdman Ballagh. *Normal Aging III: Reports from the Duke Longitudinal Studies.* Durham, NC: Duke University Press, 1985.

Pifer, Alan and Lydia Bronte. *Our Aging Society: Paradox and Promise.* New York: W. W. Norton & Company, 1986.

Prado, C. G. *Rethinking How We Age: A New View of the Aging Mind.* Contributions in Philosophy, No. 28, Westport, CT: Greenwood Press, 1986.

Schlossberg, Nancy K. *Counseling Adults in Transition.* New York: Springer Publishing Company, 1984.

Sinnott, Jan D. *Everyday Problem Solving: Theory and Applications.* New York: Praeger Publishers, 1989.

Sloan, Tod Stratton. *Deciding: Self-Deception in Life Choices.* London, UK: Methuen & Co. Ltd, 1987.

Taeuber, Cynthia M. *Sixty-Five Plus in America.* Vol. P23-178. Current Population Reports: Current Studies, ed. Nampeo McKenney. Washington, DC: U.S. Government Printing Office, 1992.

Tobin, Sheldon S. *Personhood in Advanced Old Age: Implications for Practice.* New York: Springer Publishing Company, 1991.

Vaillant, George. *Adaptation to Life.* Boston: Little, Brown and Company, 1977.

Waxman, Barbara Frey. *From the Hearth to the Open Road.* Contributions in Women's Studies, No.113, Westport, CT: Greenwood Press, 1990.

STORIES

Adams, Alice. *Second Chances.* New York: Alfred A. Knopf, 1988.

Bateson, Mary Caterine. *Composing a Life.* New York: Printing Press, 1989.

Brookner, Anita. *Fraud.* London: Jonathan Cape, 1992.

Fowler, Margaret and Priscilla McCutcheon, ed. *Songs of Experience.* New York: Ballantine Books, 1991.

Goldreich, Gloria. *Years of Dreams.* New York: Harcourt Brace Jovanovich, 1992.

Gordimer, Nadine. *A Sport of Nature.* New York: Alfred A. Knopf, 1987.

Grumbach, Doris. *Coming Into the End Zone: A Memoir.* New York: W.W. Norton & Company, 1991.

Janeway, Elizabeth. *Cross Sections: From a Decade of Change.* New York: William Morrow and Company, 1982.

Kay, Terry. *To Dance with the White Dog.* ed. Washington Square Press. New York: Pocket Books, 1990.

Kidder, Tracy. *Old Friends.* Boston: Houghton Mifflin Company, 1993.

Marshall, Paule. *Praisesong for the Widow.* New York: Penquin Books, 1983.

Martz, Sandra, ed. *When I Am An Old Woman I Shall Wear Purple.* Watsonville, CA: Papier-Mache Press, 1987.

Murdock, Maureen. *The Heroine's Journey.* Boston: Shambala Publications, 1990.

Naylor, Gloria. *Mama Day.* New York: Vintage Contempories, 1989.

Norton, Catherine Sullivan. *Life Metaphors: Stories of Ordinary Survival.* Carbondale, IL: Southern Illinois University Press, 1989.

Pilcher, Rosamunde. *The Shell Seekers.* New York: St. Martin's Press, 1987.

Sarton, May. *Endgame: A Journal of My Seventy-Ninth Year.* New York: W.W. Norton, 1992.

Tan, Amy. *The Joy Luck Club.* New York: G.P. Putnam's Sons, 1989.

Walker, Alice. *The Color Purple.* New York: Simon & Schuster, 1982.

About the Author

Patricia W. Burnham, Ph.D., is president of The Transitions Group, Inc., a research and consulting firm specializing in personal and organizational change. She has been a vice president for Chase Manhattan Bank, and an insurance and investment advisor for Nationwide Insurance Companies.

Dr. Burnham formerly managed continuing education at the Ohio State University, academic and health affairs for the Illinois Board of Higher Education, and professional development programs at Illinois State University. In recent years she has been a managing and marketing consultant to U.S. and international corporations and associations.

Dr. Burnham is a frequent speaker to business, professional, and community audiences and has published a number of professional articles and reviews. She also conducts seminars on adult transitions and serves on the boards of several organizations that manage programs for the aging.

She resides with her husband in Vermont and New York.

Life's Third Act may be ordered by sending a check for $18.95 to MasterMedia Limited, 17 East 89th Street, New York, NY 10128. Or call (800) 334-8232 or fax (212) 546-7638. Be sure to include $2 for postage and handling of the first copy, $1 for each additional copy.

MasterMedia's authors are available for speeches and seminars. Call Tony Colao at (908) 359-1612.

Other MasterMedia Books

AGING PARENTS AND YOU: *A Complete Handbook to Help You Help Your Elders Maintain a Healthy, Productive, Independent Life,* by Eugenia Anderson-Ellis, is a complete guide to providing care to aging relatives. It features practical advice and resources for adults helping their elders lead productive lives. Revised and updated. ($9.95 paper)

BALANCING ACTS! *Juggling Love, Work, Family, and Recreation,* by Susan Schiffer Stautberg and Marcia L. Worthing, provides strategies to achieve a balanced life by reordering priorities and setting realistic goals. ($12.95 paper)

BEATING THE AGE GAME: *Redefining Retirement,* by Jack and Phoebe Ballard, debunks the myth that retirement means sitting out the rest of the game. The years between 55 and 80 can be your best, say the authors, who provide ample examples of people successfully using retirement to reinvent their lives. ($12.95 paper)

BEYOND SUCCESS: *How Volunteer Service Can Help You Begin Making a Life Instead of Just a Living,* by John J. Raynolds III and Eleanor Raynolds, C.B.E., is a unique how-to book targeted at business and professional people considering volunteer work, senior citizens who wish to fill leisure time meaningfully, and students trying out career options. ($9.95 paper, $19.95 cloth)

THE BIG APPLE BUSINESS AND PLEASURE GUIDE: *501 Ways To Work Smarter, Play Harder, and Live Better in New York City,* by

Muriel Siebert and Susan Kleinman, offers visitors and New Yorkers alike advice on how to do business in the city as well as how to enjoy its attractions. ($9.95 paper)

BREATHING SPACE: *Living and Working at a Comfortable Pace in a Sped-Up Society,* by Jeff Davidson, helps readers to handle information and activity overload, in order to gain greater control over their lives. ($10.95 paper)

CITIES OF OPPORTUNITY: *Finding the Best Way to Work, Live, and Prosper in the 1990s and Beyond,* by Dr. John Tepper Martin, explores the job and living options for the next decade and into the next century. This consumer guide and handbook, written by one of the world's experts on cities, selects and features forty-six American cities and metropolitan areas. ($13.95 paper, $24.95 cloth)

THE CONFIDENCE FACTOR: *How Self-Esteem Can Change Your Life,* by Dr. Judith Briles, is based on a nationwide survey of six thousand men and women. Briles explores why women so often feel a lack of self-confidence and have a poor opinion of themselves. She offers step-by-step advice on becoming the person you want to be. ($12.95 paper, $18.95 cloth)

DARE TO CONFRONT! *How To Intervene When Someone You Care About Has a Drug or Alcohol Problem,* by Bob Wright and Deborah George Wright, shows the reader how to use the step-by-step methods of professional interventionists to motivate drug-dependent people to accept help they need. ($17.95 cloth)

THE DOLLARS AND SENSE OF DIVORCE: *The Financial Guide for Women,* by Dr. Judith Briles, is the first book to combine the legal hurdles by planning finances before, during, and after divorce. ($10.95 paper)

THE ENVIRONMENTAL GARDENER: *The Solution to Pollution for Lawns and Gardens,* by Laurence Sombke, focuses on what each of us can do to protect our endangered plant life. A practical source book and shopping guide. ($8.95 paper)

FINANCIAL SAVVY FOR WOMEN: *A Money Book for Women of All Ages,* by Dr. Judith Briles, divides a woman's monetary life span into six phases, discusses specific issues to be addressed at each stage, and demonstrates how to create a sound money plan. ($15.00 paper)

FLIGHT PLAN FOR LIVING: *The Art of Self-Encouragement,* by Patrick O'Dooley, is a life guide organized like a pilot's checklist, to ensure you'll be flying "clear on top" throughout your life. ($17.95 cloth)

GLORIOUS ROOTS: *Recipes for Healthy, Tasty Vegetables,* by Laurence Sombke, celebrates the taste, texture, and versatility of root vegetables. Contains recipes for appetizers, soups, stews, and baked, broiled, and stir-fried dishes—even desserts. ($12.95 paper)

HOT HEALTH-CARE CAREERS, by Margaret T. McNally, R.N., and Phyllis Schneider, provides readers everything they need to know about training for and getting jobs in a rewarding field where professionals are always in demand. ($10.95 paper)

HOW TO GET WHAT YOU WANT FROM ALMOST ANYBODY, by T. Scott Gross, shows how to get great service, negotiate better prices, and always get what you pay for. ($9.95 paper)

KIDS WHO MAKE A DIFFERENCE, by Joyce M. Roché and Marie Rodriguez, is an inspiring document of how today's toughest challenges are being met by teenagers and kids, whose courage and creativity enables them to find practical solutions! ($8.95 paper, with photos)

THE LIVING HEART BRAND NAME SHOPPER'S GUIDE, by Michael E. DeBakey, M.D., Antonio M. Gotto, Jr., M.D., Lynne W. Scott, M.A., R.D./L.D., and John P. Foreyt, Ph.D., lists brand name products low in fat, saturated fatty acids, and cholesterol. Revised edition. ($14.95 paper)

THE LIVING HEART GUIDE TO EATING OUT, by Michael E. DeBakey, Antonio M. Gotto, Jr., and Lynne W. Scott, is an essential handbook for people who want to maintain a health-conscious diet when dining in all types of restaurants. ($9.95 paper)

THE LOYALTY FACTOR: *Building Trust in Today's Workplace,* by Carol Kinsey Goman, Ph.D., offers techniques for restoring commitment and loyalty in the workplace. ($9.95 paper)

MAKING YOUR DREAMS COME TRUE: *A Plan For Easily Discovering and Achieving the Life You Want,* by Marcia Wieder, introduces an easy, unique, and practical technique for defining, pursuing, and realizing your career and life interests. Filled with stories of real people and helpful exercises, plus a personal workbook. ($9.95 paper)

MANAGING IT ALL: *Time-Saving Ideas for Career, Family, Relationships, and Self,* by Beverly Treuille and Susan Stautberg, is written for women juggling careers and families. With interviews of more than two hundred career women, this book contains many humorous anecdotes on saving time and improving the quality of life. ($9.95 paper)

MANAGING YOUR CHILD'S DIABETES, by Robert Wood Johnson IV, Sale Johnson, Casey Johnson, and Susan Kleinman, brings help to families trying to understand diabetes and control its effects. ($10.95 paper)

MANAGING YOUR PSORIASIS, by Nicholas J. Lowe, M.D., is an innovative manual that couples scientific research and encouraging support, with an emphasis on how patients can take charge of their health. ($10.95 paper, $17.95 cloth)

MANN FOR ALL SEASONS: *Wit and Wisdom from* The Washington Post's *Judy Mann,* shows the columnist at her best as she writes about women, families, and the impact and politics of the women's revolution. ($9.95 paper, $19.95 cloth)

MIND YOUR OWN BUSINESS: *And Keep it in the Family*, by Marcy Syms, CEO of Syms Corp, is an effective guide for any organization facing the toughest step in managing a family business— making the transition to the new generation. ($12.95 paper, $18.95 cloth)

OFFICE BIOLOGY: *Why Tuesday Is the Most Productive Day and Other Relevant Facts for Survival in the Workplace,* by Edith Weiner and Arnold Brown, teaches how in the '90s and beyond we will be expected to work smarter, take better control of our health, adapt to advancing technology, and improve our lives in ways that are not too costly or resource-intensive. ($12.95 paper, $21.95 cloth)

ON TARGET: *Enhance Your Life and Advance Your Career,* by Jeri Sedlar and Rick Miners, is a neatly woven tapestry of insights on career and life issues gathered from audiences across the country. This feedback has been crystallized into a highly readable guide for exploring who you are and how to go about getting what you want. ($11.95 paper)

OUT THE ORGANIZATION: *New Career Opportunities for the 1990s,* by Robert and Madeleine Swain, is written for the millions of Americans whose jobs are no longer safe, whose companies are not loyal, and who face futures of uncertainty, provides advice on finding a new job or starting your own business. (Revised $12.95 paper, $17.95 cloth)

THE OUTDOOR WOMAN: *A Handbook to Adventure,* by Patricia Hubbard and Stan Wass, details the lives of adventurous women and offers their ideas on how you can incorporate exciting outdoor experiences into your life. ($14.95 paper)

PAIN RELIEF: *How to Say No to Acute and Chronic Pain,* by Dr. Jane Cowles, offers a step-by-step plan for assessing pain and communicating it to your doctor, and explains the importance of having a pain plan before undergoing any medical or surgical treatment; includes "The Pain Patient's Bill of Rights," and a reusable pain assessment chart. ($22.95 paper)

POSITIVELY OUTRAGEOUS SERVICE: *New and Easy Ways To Win Customers for Life,* by T. Scott Gross, identifies what '90s consumers really want and how business can develop effective marketing strategies to answer those needs. ($14.95 paper)

POSITIVELY OUTRAGEOUS SERVICE AND SHOWMANSHIP, by T. Scott Gross, reveals the secrets of adding personality to any product or service and offers a wealth of nontraditional marketing techniques employed by top showmen, from car dealers to restaurateurs, amusement park operators to evangelists. ($12.95 paper)

THE PREGNANCY AND MOTHERHOOD DIARY: *Planning the First Year of Your Second Career,* by Susan Schiffer Stautberg, is only undated appointment diary that shows how to manage pregnancy and career. ($12.95 spiralbound)

REAL BEAUTY...REAL WOMEN: *A Handbook for Making the Best of Your Own Good Looks,* by Kathleen Walas, International Beauty and Fashion Director of Avon Products, Inc., offers expert advice on beauty and fashion for women of all ages and ethnic backgrounds. ($19.95 paper)

REAL LIFE 101: *The Graduate's Guide To Survival,* by Susan Kleinman, supplies welcome advice to those facing "real life" for the first time, focusing on work, money, health, and how to deal with freedom and responsibility. Revised. ($9.95 paper)

ROSEY GRIER'S ALL-AMERICAN HEROES: *Multicultural Success Stories,* by Roosevelt "Rosey" Grier, is a candid collection of profiles of prominent African Americans, Latins, Asians, and Native Americans who revealed how they achieved public acclaim and personal success. ($9.95 paper, with photos)

SELLING YOURSELF: *How To Be the Competent, Confident Person You Really Are!* by Kathy Thebo and Joyce Newman, is an inspirational primer for anyone seeking to project a positive image. Drawing on experience, their own and others', these entrepreneurs offer simple techniques that can add up to big successes. ($11.95 paper)

SHOCKWAVES: *The Global Impact of Sexual Harassment,* by Susan L. Webb, examines the problem of sexual harassment today in every kind of workplace around the world. Practical and well-researched, this manual provides the most recent information available, including legal changes in progress. ($11.95 paper, $19.95 cloth)

SIDE-BY-SIDE STRATEGIES*: How Two-Career Couples Can Thrive in the '90s,* by Jane Hershey Cuozzo and S. Diane Graham, describes how to learn the difference between competing with a spouse and become a supportive power partner. Published in hardcover as *Power Partners.* ($10.95 paper, $19.95 cloth)

THE SOLUTION TO POLLUTION: *101 Things You Can Do To Clean Up Your Environment,* by Laurence Sombke, offers step-by-step techniques on how to conserve more energy, start a recycling center, choose a biodegradable product, and even proceed with individual clean-up projects. ($7.95 paper)

THE SOLUTION TO POLLUTION IN THE WORKPLACE, by Laurence Sombke, Terry M. Robertson, and Elliot M. Kaplan, offers everything employees need to know about cleaning up their workplace, including recycling, using energy efficiently, conserving water, and buying nontoxic supplies. ($9.95 paper)

SOMEONE ELSE'S SON, by Alan A. Winter, explores the parent-child bond in a contemporary novel of lost identities, family secrets, and relationships gone awry. Eighteen years after bringing their first son home from the hospital, Trish and Brad Hunter discover they are not his biological parents. ($18.95 cloth)

STEP FORWARD: *Sexual Harassment in the Workplace*, by Susan L. Webb, presents the facts for dealing with sexual harassment on the job. ($9.95 paper)

THE STEPPARENT CHALLENGE: *A Primer For Making It Work,* by Stephen J. Williams, Ph.D., offers insight into the many aspects of step relationships—from financial issues to lifestyle changes to differences in race or religion that affect the whole family. ($13.95 paper)

STRAIGHT TALK ON WOMEN'S HEALTH: *How to Get the Health Care You Deserve,* by Janice Teal and Phyllis Schneider, is destined to become a health-care "bible." Devoid of confusing medical jargon, it offers a wealth of resources, including contact lists of healthlines and women's medical centers. ($14.95 paper)

TAKING CONTROL OF YOUR LIFE: *The Secrets of Successful Enterprising Women,* by Gail Blanke and Kathleen Walas, is based on the authors' professional experience with Avon Products' Women of Enterprise Awards, given each year to outstanding female entrepreneurs; it offers a plan to help you gain control over your life, plus business tips as well as beauty and lifestyle information. ($17.95 cloth)

TEAMBUILT: *Making Teamwork Work,* by Mark Sanborn, teaches businesses how to increase productivity, without increasing resources or expenses, by building teamwork among employees. ($12.95 paper, $19.95 cloth)

A TEEN'S GUIDE TO BUSINESS: *The Secrets to a Successful Enterprise,* by Linda Menzies, Oren S. Jenkins, and Rick R. Fisher, provides solid information about starting your own business or working for one. ($7.95 paper)

TWENTYSOMETHING: *Managing & Motivating Today's New Work Force,* by Lawrence J. Bradford, Ph.D., and Claire Raines, M.A., examines the work orientation of the younger generation and offers managers practical advice for understanding and supervising their young employees. ($12.95 paper, $22.95 cloth)

WHAT KIDS LIKE TO DO, by Edward Stautberg, Gail Wubbenhorst, Atiya Easterling, and Phyllis Schneider, is a handy guide for parents, grandparents, and baby sitters. Written by kids for kids, this is an easy-to-read, generously illustrated primer for teaching families how to make every day more fun. ($7.95 paper)